Addressing Violence, Abuse and Oppression

Everyone working in health and social care is at one point or another confronted by violent behaviour and its consequences. *Addressing Violence, Abuse and Oppression* provides a broad overview of violence in relation to a range of groups and areas that involve human service professionals.

Adopting an international perspective, this book looks at the ways in which violence, abuse and oppression can be clearly associated with power imbalances which are often gendered and which are covertly or overtly manifested at a range of levels including the interpersonal as well as the organizational and the political. It explores debates and challenges with regard to theoretical orientations, policy frameworks and how power imbalances intersect with a range of influencing factors including gender, poverty, indigenous/ethnic issues, class and sexuality.

Examining the implications for human service professionals, each chapter of *Addressing Violence, Abuse and Oppression* provides an historical overview, explores theoretical perspectives, examines specific policy and practice contexts, appraises the contribution from research and assesses the impact for individuals and groups.

Barbara Fawcett is Professor of Social Work and Policy Studies at the University of Sydney.

Fran Waugh is a senior lecturer in the Social Work and Policy Studies programmes in the Faculty of Education and Social Work at the University of Sydney.

Addressing Violence, Abuse and Oppression

Debates and challenges

Edited by
**Barbara Fawcett and
Fran Waugh**

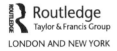

LONDON AND NEW YORK

First published 2008
by Routledge
2 Park Square, Milton Park, Abingdon Oxon OX14 4RN

Simultaneously published in the USA and Canada
by Routledge
711 Third Avenue, New York, NY 10017

Routledge is an imprint of the Taylor & Francis Group, an informa business

© 2008 Selection and editorial matter Barbara Fawcett and Fran Waugh;
individual chapters the contributors

Typeset in Times New Roman by
Book Now Ltd

British Library Cataloguing in Publication Data
A catalogue record for this book is available from the British Library

Library of Congress Cataloging in Publication Data
A catalog record for this book has been requested

ISBN10: 0–415–42263–9 (hbk)
ISBN10: 0–415–42264–7 (pbk)
ISBN10: 0–203–93771–6 (ebk)

ISBN13: 978–0–415–42263–5 (hbk)
ISBN13: 978–0–415–42264–2 (pbk)
ISBN13: 978–0–203–93771–6 (ebk)

Contents

vi *Contents*

Contributors

Maurice Hanlon is a lecturer at the Australian Catholic University based at the Strathfield campus in Sydney. He spent eight years working in the field in the United Kingdom before becoming a lecturer in social work and social policy at Bradford College. He joined the Australian Catholic University in 2006. His research interests include social work and ethics, disability, gender studies and anti-oppressive anti-discriminatory practice.

Deborah Hart worked as a social worker in the Australian Government income support and employment services arena for sixteen years before taking up a position in the Social Work and Policy Studies programme at the University of Sydney. During Deborah's direct social work practice experience in the Department of Social Security and Centrelink, she was required to work on a daily basis with people from diverse backgrounds who were struggling with the lived experience of poverty and with the emotional and material challenges of escaping violence, abuse and oppression. Deborah is currently engaged in doctoral research that looks at the impact on Australian social workers of administering an increasingly stringent welfare reform environment within a rapidly changing public service context.

Jude Irwin is an Associate Professor in the Faculty of Education and Social Work at the University of Sydney. Her teaching, research, practice and policy interests span a number of areas including violence against women, children and young people, discrimination against gay men and lesbians and professional practice supervision. Jude Irwin is a member of the NSW Child Death Review Team and the NSW Ombudsman's Child Death Advisory Group. She has published widely, including four co-edited books, numerous journal articles and several public reports.

Lesley Laing is a Senior Lecturer in Social Work and Policy Studies at the University of Sydney. She is a social worker who has worked in direct service delivery, policy, training and research in the fields of community health, child and adolescent mental health, child protection and violence against women. In 2000, she established the Australian Domestic and Family Violence Clearinghouse at the University of NSW. Prior to this, she was Director of the

New South Wales Education Centre Against Violence where she established statewide training programmes and developed educational resources for health workers on adult and child sexual assault, domestic violence, and child protection programmes. She is currently involved in research on coordinated responses to domestic violence; post-separation violence against women and children; domestic violence and women's mental health; and treatment effectiveness with young people who have been sexually abused.

Denise Lynch has worked as a Lecturer at the University of Sydney for the past ten years. Her areas of interest are child protection and refugee and asylum seeking children. She has conducted research on asylum seeking children and families in Sydney with a grant from the Don Chipp Foundation. Her practice history is in child welfare and child protection in NSW, where she has held senior management positions.

Lorna McNamara has spent twenty years in direct work in mental health, drug and alcohol and women and youth services. She has been with the Education Centre Against Violence since 1994 delivering training programmes on sexual assault and domestic violence in the mental health sector. Lorna played a pivotal role in research on the sexual assault of women in mental health services, which subsequently led to the development of sexual safety policy for that sector. She has been Director of the Education Centre Against Violence since 2002, and has worked alongside the Aboriginal training team restructuring the service to incorporate the Aboriginal Community Matters Advisory Group in decision-making processes within the Centre.

Karen Menzies is an Aboriginal woman from the Wonnarua people of the Hunter Valley, NSW. Karen has an extensive background in child protection, education, health and human rights. She currently works as an Education and Training Consultant. Karen also has a Conjoint Social Work Lecturer position with the University of Newcastle.

Lindsey Napier is Pro Dean in the Faculty of Education and Social Work at the University of Sydney. She co-edited *Breakthroughs in Practice: Theorising Critical Moments in Social Work* with Jan Fook. Her current research focuses on social work in dying, death and bereavement, on good practice in community care for people with dementia and on access to appropriate services for women experiencing both mental illness and domestic violence.

Agi O'Hara, a Lecturer in psychology in Social Work and Policy Studies in the Faculty of Education and Social Work at the University of Sydney, is a registered psychologist with many years of experience working with individuals, couples and groups. She provides clinical supervision to other human service professionals and is the co-author of *Skills for Human Service Practice: Working with Individuals, Groups and Communities*, published by Oxford University Press. Agi O'Hara's teaching specialties include counselling, suicide prevention, depression, child abuse, domestic violence and enhanced learning through flexible learning strategies. Her research interests include mentoring disadvantaged youth and professional ethics.

Ruth Phillips is a Senior Lecturer in Social Work and Policy Studies at the University of Sydney. Prior to completing her PhD degree at the University of New South Wales in 2001, she worked in the Western Australian State Government as a policy officer and ministerial policy adviser in the areas of community services, social policy and women's policy. Her areas of research include third sector studies, social policy and the welfare state. She has previous journal articles and book chapters published on all of her research interests, including the relationships between feminism and Australian domestic violence policy.

Rosalie Pockett has recently joined the academic staff in Social Work and Policy Studies at the University of Sydney. Prior to this she was a director of social work services in hospital and health services in western Sydney and a senior social work practitioner. Her research interests include health and hospital practice, the occupational culture of social work and developing practice-based research in the field. Her most recent publications include: 'Learning from each other: the social work role as an integrated part of the hospital disaster response', *Social Work in Health Care*, 43 (2/3) (2006): 131–49; 'Staying in hospital social work', *Social Work in Health Care*, 36 (3) (2003): 1–23.

Margot Rawsthorne is currently employed as a Lecturer (Community Development) in Social Work and Policy Studies at the University of Sydney. She has considerable expertise in undertaking qualitative research, particularly with non-traditional research participants. She views qualitative research as a means of giving marginalized groups a voice. Over recent years her research has highlighted the issues of sole parents, Aboriginal women, rural women, women from non-English speaking backgrounds and vulnerable families. In 2006 she undertook a research project with lesbian parents. She has an extensive network of contacts in community services, having worked as a community worker in Western Sydney for fifteen years.

Zita Weber is a lecturer in Social Work and Policy Studies at The University of Sydney. Prior to entering academia, Zita worked in a number of mental health and rehabilitation settings. Zita teaches in both the undergraduate and graduate Social Work programme. Her research areas include mental health, loss and grief, migrant and women's issues. In addition to published papers, Zita is the author of four books for the general public: *Back from the Blues*, *Out of the Blues*, *Good Grief* and *The Best Years of a Woman's Life* and co-author of *Skills for Human Service Practice: Working with Individuals, Groups and Communities*, published by Oxford University Press.

Editors

Fran Waugh is a Senior Lecturer in Social Work and Policy Studies at the University of Sydney. Fran has an extensive practice background working in community health, family support and in child protection in both health and welfare settings. Fran is an active researcher and her focus on practice research in areas of Australian national priorities such as child emotional abuse, child protection and domestic violence, paediatric palliative care and older people with dementia, is drawn from rigorous and often difficult engagement with these vulnerable and at-risk groups. In addition to her undergraduate and postgraduate teaching responsibilities, Fran has participated in Field Education since her academic appointment in 2000.

Barbara Fawcett is Professor of Social Work and Policy Studies in the Faculty of Education and Social Work at the University of Sydney. Previously she was Head of the Department of Social Sciences and Humanities at the University of Bradford. She has considerable professional as well as academic experience. Her research interests focus on women and violence, disability, mental health, action research and postmodern feminism. Previous books include:

Fawcett, B., Featherstone, B., Hearn, J. and Toft, C. (eds) (1996) *Violence and Gender Relations: Theories and Interventions*. London: Sage.

Fawcett, B., Featherstone, B., Fook, J. and Rossiter, A. (eds) (2000) *Research and Practice in Social Work: Postmodern Feminist Perspectives*. London: Routledge.

Fawcett, B. (2000) *Feminist Perspectives on Disability*. Harlow: Prentice Hall.

Fawcett, B., Featherstone, B. and Goddard, J. (2004) *Contemporary Child Care Policy and Practice*. Basingstoke: Palgrave.

Fawcett, B. and Karban, K. (2005) *Contemporary Mental Health: Theory, Policy and Practice*. London: Routledge.

Acknowledgements

We would like to thank all the contributors to the book for their commitment and enthusiasm. We would particularly like to thank Agi O'Hara for her patience and expertise in compiling the bibliography. We would also like to thank Jan Larbalestier, Moya Turner and Kate and Sophie Hanlon for their encouragement and support.

We would also like to acknowledge the women of Mother of Mercy Women's House, Cerro Candela, Lima, Peru, who are inspiring in their solidarity to overcome oppression and create a better future for their children and their community. And to Joan Doyle, Jackie Ford and Trish McDermott who listen with their hearts and act with their lives in striving for social justice.

1   Introduction

This book focuses on violence, abuse and oppression and explores debates and challenges with regard to policy frameworks and influencing factors such as poverty, status and age. It adopts an international perspective and critically examines the implications of policy and practice for different groupings of people in different contexts, taking full account of aspects such as ethnicity, indigenous issues, class and sexuality.

Definitions of violence, abuse and oppression vary. Abuse and oppression can be regarded as manifestations of violence, with violence being broadly defined to include psychological, emotional and economic as well as physical aspects. A related, but differing approach is to focus on the ways in which these three areas are interconnected and intermeshed. Alternatively abuse and oppression can be considered separately in order to draw attention to the ways in which structural power imbalances can adversely affect marginalized groups in public and private settings. The chapters in this book both recognize and relate to these varying perspectives, but a common theme throughout is to both understand and respond to violence, abuse and oppression as social processes with social consequences. These are in turn intricately associated with the position of the person or group undertaking the defining. As a result, throughout the book understandings of violence, abuse and oppression are continually interrogated in relation to the specific area being discussed.

Gender has to feature strongly in any discussion of violence, abuse and oppression. Whether referring to what has variously been termed domestic violence, intimate partner violence or violence to a known other, or to forms of public or state violence, statistics demonstrate that although women are perpetrators, and not all men are violent, far more men commit violent acts than women. As a result there is a clear focus in this book on the operation and reproduction of gendered power imbalances at individual and social levels. The chapters have also been informed by the historical development of the various feminisms (for example, radical, liberal, socialist, ecological, postmodern) as well as by contemporary contributions and these have been used to explore a wide range of issues relating to violence, oppression and abuse.

As violence, abuse and oppression are clearly associated with power imbalances, which can be covertly or overtly manifested at a range of levels and which include the interpersonal as well as the organizational and the political, it is recognized that analysis of theory, policy and practice, whilst imperative, has to be accompanied by action. What this is and how it is played out will vary according to context, but the ways in which those working in the human services operate both strategically and operationally is significant. In order to facilitate action, all of the contributors to the book examine and explore the implications for human service providers of their analysis and highlight key pointers for further change.

Violence, abuse and oppression have an international resonance and in this book emphasis is placed on maintaining an international relevance whilst also ensuring that there is a focus on specific countries to provide examples or to illustrate the arguments and points being made. The countries referred to include western nations such as Australia, the United Kingdom, Canada and the USA as well as countries such as Malawi, Bangladesh and Uganda. This broad span facilitates international comparisons and highlights the very different concerns held by different groups. Clearly there are commonalities, but there are also specific issues which require attention.

The book has been divided into three parts. The first concentrates on violence, abuse and oppression as they affect 'women' and 'men' and explores links and associations between these areas and poverty and indigenous issues. Barbara Fawcett, in the chapter on women and violence, looks at understandings of 'domestic violence' or intimate partner violence and the associations which have been made between violence and abuse. She considers the effect of violence on women's health and argues that although domestic violence is intrinsically related to gendered power imbalances which are represented differently in varying social and cultural contexts, the view that violence is inevitable, even when tacitly sanctioned by social, cultural and economic practices, is not the case. She emphasizes the importance of zero tolerance campaigns, but highlights the need to explore the ways in which gendered power imbalances foster intimate partner violence in some contexts but not in others. Maurice Hanlon focuses on men and violence. He interrogates the theoretical perspectives which have been put forward to account for gendered violence and examines key features from the burgeoning men and masculinities literature over the past decade before exploring the issues associated with violent men and fathering. Deborah Hart appraises the connections which can be made between poverty and violence in a global context. She explores the challenges faced by people who live in poverty to escape from relationships dominated by violence, abuse and oppression before moving on to address a number of specific questions. These include the ways in which the experience of violence might be different for people living in poverty, how current and emerging social and economic policies and practices maintain oppressive relationships of dependence, and the social and economic policies and practices that promote opportunities to escape violence, abuse and oppression. The chapter on aboriginal issues and violence focuses on Australia. Aboriginal communities experience violence at rates far in excess of the wider community. This violence can only be understood within the context of the historical and traumatic experiences endured by Aboriginal people as a result of unjust and oppressive state policies and practices. These are exemplified by child welfare policies that resulted in the forcible removal of generations of Aboriginal children from their families. Even today, as evidenced by Federal Government incursions into the Northern Territory, Aboriginal people are subject to insensitive and oppressive policies and practices which erode, rather than build on and further develop, existing strengths. This chapter explores the ways in which Aboriginal people are speaking out against the violence in their communities and the strategies they are employing to rebuild Aboriginal society.

Part II starts off with Ruth Phillips exploring feminism(s) and domestic violence within national policy contexts. This chapter examines the role and character of a range of national responses to domestic violence and makes links to wider political and social transformations. These include consideration of the impact of the women's movement, the concomitant backlash, global social policy issues which focus on human rights, and the contemporary political rift between the West and the Islamic world which raises issues about interventions regarding violence against women across diverse cultures. This chapter is followed by Lesley Laing's appraisal of 'violence', criminal justice and the law. Within the context of intimate partner violence, Laing examines legal responses and both past and current challenges. She employs feminist analyses to explore the extent to which legal remedies have achieved the core goals of domestic violence policy which are increasing the safety of women and holding the perpetrators accountable. She notes that using the law has proved more complex and difficult than originally anticipated and she appraises the challenges that have arisen in order to chart the way forward. Jude Irwin explores violence within lesbian relationships and examines how the development of discourses surrounding domestic violence have influenced and produced particular understandings of intimate partner violence between lesbians. She draws on stories of lesbians who have experienced intimate partner violence to show that while they may encounter similar forms of abuse in their relationships to those encountered by heterosexual women, the heteronormative discursive constitutions of intimate partner violence both generate and limit understandings and responses to such violence, accentuating its obscurity. Margot Rawsthorne draws from an ecological approach to review the situation of rural women. Contrary to stereotypical images of rural communities, Rawsthorne maintains that multiple bonded ties create barriers to women gaining or seeking support to escape violence. This results from an interplay of personal, situational, and socio-cultural factors which not only makes violence more likely, but also continues to perpetuate the silence and inadequate response to this violence.

Part III Three is concerned with the impact of violence, abuse and oppression on different groupings of people. It is accepted that these groupings cannot be viewed as homogeneous, but significant features are highlighted and interrogated. Fran Waugh's chapter on violence against children within the family examines the theoretical perspectives, the policy underpinnings and the practice implications of measures used in countries such as Australia, the United Kingdom and the United States of America to combat this emotive and highly political area. Key concepts related to risk, protection and resilience are explored and challenges, which include developing policies and practices which are evidence-based and are cognizant of the complexities of children's and parents' lives as well as the need for the meaningful participation of children and parents in the development of effectual partnerships, are appraised.

Denise Lynch, using Australia as a case study, argues that structural violence is being perpetrated against asylum seeker children following arrival in their country of destination. She illustrates this argument by providing evidence relating to the difficulties experienced with regard to health, education, housing and poverty. She draws attention to how this form of structural violence and oppression, caused in some part by their unresolved legal status, results in children being unable to develop and form an identity or a sense of belonging with their new country. In consequence, she maintains that perceptions of Australia as a country, where children and families are given a 'fair go' is questionable. Zita Weber concentrates on the contentious arena of mental health and violence. She explores the rise of the contemporary collective movement of consumers of mental health services and assesses the importance of this in challenging the history of past institutional and professional violence, abuse and oppression. She draws from past and present scenarios to examine entrenched controversies and to formulate a vision of enabling policies and practices. Agi O'Hara looks at suicide as the most severe form of violence against the self. She recognizes that an individual may be prompted to take this course of action as a result of organizational, individual and/or routinized acts of abuse and oppression and explores the various understandings which have been put forward, the connections which can be made with self-harm, and reviews associated motivational features, 'risk' factors and policy aspects.

Barbara Fawcett provides an historical overview of how disability has been both understood and responded to and interrogates conceptualizations of disability and the links and association which can be made between these and issues concerning violence, abuse and oppression. She appraises the concept of 'vulnerability' and argues that assessment and protection measures can further constrain rather than promote wellbeing and security. Lindsey Napier and Fran Waugh identify the different ways in which older people have been characterized with respect to their experience of violence, abuse and oppression. They critically review oppressive perceptions and make links between theory, policy and practice before discussing possible ways forward. Rosalie Pockett interrogates controversies relating to human service professionals, violence and the workplace. In this, she critically examines debates surrounding the incidence, measurement and cost of workplace violence, causative factors and the current discourse on the management, containment and elimination of workplace violence. Finally, in the concluding chapter, the key themes raised in all the chapters relating to the multifaceted and complex nature of violence, abuse and oppression and the ways in which violence, abuse and oppression intersect with aspects such as age, ethnicity and the operation of gendered power imbalances are appraised. The implications for human service professionals are also re-emphasized and summarized and ways forward are considered.

Part I

Lenses for understanding

Framing debates within violence, abuse and oppression

2 Women and violence

Barbara Fawcett

Domestic violence is a global issue which resonates throughout society. Its manifestation in social relations reflects gendered power imbalances and social divisions. The impact of domestic violence is wide ranging and considerable. It affects the safety as well as the health and wellbeing of individuals. It also negatively influences individual and social resilience and the capacity to build and maintain strong communities.In this chapter, a number of key areas will be examined. These include an examination of definitions and explanations of domestic violence and an appraisal of associations which have been made between violence and abuse. As part of the discussion multi-country links between women's health and domestic violence will be explored and matters associated with professional responsibility and responses will be considered.

As a starting point, it has to be recognized that domestic violence can include violence between directly or indirectly related family members as well as intimate partner violence. The focus of this chapter is on domestic violence defined as intimate partner violence and this takes place between partners or former partners and includes violence perpetrated by men against women, by women against men and violence which occurs in same-sex relationships. However, although domestic violence perpetrated by women against men is gaining currency as a social issue, available research and statistics consistently show that the predominant form of domestic violence relates to violence towards women by men. In the European Union, for example, 25 per cent of all violent crimes reported involve a man assaulting his wife or partner (European Parliament, 2005). In the United Kingdom, domestic violence accounts for 31 per cent of all violence against women (Home Office, 2006) and in Australia, 1.1 million women experience violence by a partner both during and after the relationship (Carrington and Phillips, 2003). With regard to this latter example, it is important to acknowledge that as the population of Australia is approximately 20 million people, this constitutes a significant figure. It is also notable that intimate partner violence cuts across class divisions, age related factors and ethnic distinctions.

In relation to what domestic or intimate partner violence can be seen to incorporate, it is pertinent that whilst some commentators focus particularly on direct physical violence (for example, Mullender, 1996), others emphasize that domestic violence can be wider ranging, incorporating emotional and sexual elements, threats and forms of humiliation and control (Hearn, 1996; Hearn and Whitehead, 2006). Hearn (1996) drawing from his own research, highlights how male violators variously deny, rationalize, excuse or belittle their actions. In contrast, he found that for women, often the more wide ranging elements were reported as being the most damaging. The women who participated in the research also emphasized how the lack of control over the initiation of their partner's behaviour, the subsequent interaction and their uncertainty about the outcome, increased the intensity and fear of the violent encounter for them.

With regard to the relationship between violence and abuse, it is notable that some commentators maintain that these areas have to be viewed as separate (for example, Hague and Malos, 1993), whilst others regard the two as intermeshed (for example, Humphries and Joseph, 2004). There is also an argument for 'abuse' and 'abusive acts' to be defined as violence with 'violence' being seen to incorporate physical violence, emotional violence, sexual violence as well as maltreatment (Wang Lih-Rong, 2006). The Victorian Health Promotion Foundation (2004) reports violence 'can occur on a continuum of economic, psychological and sexual violence' which spans all cultural and socio-economic groups (Victorian Health Promotion Foundation 2004: 5). Clearly the perspectives presented, can be seen to reflect the orientation of the commentator and the context in which they are writing or undertaking research. However, a major point of difference is that whilst the term 'domestic violence' or 'intimate partner violence' emphasizes violence in the home and between partners, the term 'abuse', tends to create associations with a wider range of settings, individuals and groups. These incorporate residential or resource centres, as well as private homes, and include children, older people and disabled adults.

A discussion looking at those factors which can be seen to constitute abuse, as with definitions of violence, can be very wide ranging. 'Abuse' can incorporate physical abuse, sexual abuse, financial or material abuse and exploitation, involuntary isolation and confinement, as well as various forms of psychological abuse. This in turn can include emotional abuse as well as verbal abuse, harassment and being subject to controlling behaviour. As highlighted above, systemic and discriminatory forms of abuse, as numerous scandals in different countries have shown, demonstrates how professional workers can both inflict and be drawn into perpetrating institutionally systemic forms of abuse in both private and publicly funded settings.

Oppression, as with 'violence' and 'abuse' has been defined in a number of different ways. However, an operational definition is to view oppression as persistent negative discrimination across a wide range of areas which connect and intersect and which operate at institutional as well as at individual levels. Gendered power imbalances will be explored later in this chapter, but at this point it is useful to explore the explanations of violence, abuse and oppressive behaviour which have been put forward.

In relation to explanations of domestic violence and abuse, commentators have sought to explain violence to a known other or domestic violence in a variety of different ways and these explanations are not mutually exclusive. There are those interpretations which have focused on individual pathology. These tend to regard the perpetrator as either having a personality disorder, or a major problem related to alcohol or drug abuse, or having learnt this behaviour as part of a cyclical process where violent behaviour is transmitted through the generations. All of these explanations can be associated with the tendency to view violence in the home as a private matter. These can also be associated with a reluctance to intervene and to the attribution of a degree of responsibility towards the women who choose to remain in violent relationships.

Other explanations draw attention to social causational factors such as economic, social and familial stressors. It is notable, for example, that during the 2006 World Cup matches in the United Kingdom, significantly more cases of domestic violence were reported to the police than for the same period in 2005.[1] Associated with stressor arguments, there can be an accompanying rationale which links the removal of the stressors with the removal of the problem. However, feminist perspectives (and as Fawcett (2006) points out there is not just one feminist perspective, but a number) highlight that solutions are not so straightforward and draw attention to the pervasive effects of gendered power imbalances. Feminist orientations emphasize that domestic violence or intimate partner violence was largely regarded as an aspect of taken for granted social practices that took place in private settings and was attributable to the pathology of those involved until second wave feminism in the 1980s started to explore issues relating to gender, power and socio-political factors (Dobash, Dobash, Cavanagh and Lewis, 2000; Partnership Against Domestic Violence, 2003). Feminist perspectives regard gendered power imbalances and the expectations of obedience, duty, fidelity and submission which they can create as constituting the problem and the importance of challenging these in both public and private spheres is correspondingly promoted. Gao Jianguo and Li Qin (2006) in an exploration of community perspectives with regard to domestic violence in mainland China point to how 'societies of male superiority', traditional family values, community constraints and political expediency, serve to both downplay and hide domestic violence. Hung Suet-lin (2006), looking at the situation with regard to women coming from mainland China to Hong Kong as a result of marriage arrangements, highlights how domestic violence is often explained in terms of an unhealthy style of communication, poor socialization and learnt violent responses to frustration and personality problems. She stresses that gendered approaches which do not either address sexual politics in the family or structurally orientated social divisions related to race and ethnicity, serve to individualize and fragment responses and to dilute the message of anti-violence campaigns.

There are also explanations which associate violence in the home with an increase in violence in society generally. These point to the influence of the media,

1 West Yorkshire police in Wakefield reported 313 arrests for domestic violence offences compared with 161 during the same period in 2005. Similarly, South Wales police reported that domestic violence incidents in June 2006 were 36.8 per cent higher than the numbers recorded in June 2005 (Home Office, 2006).

film and television and to the erosion of internal and external practices of surveillance and social control. Following on from this, there are those who make links with global state violence (the war on terror, for example, in the name of a particular version of democracy) and violence being perpetuated within societies, within communities and within the domestic sphere.

The actions of governments have also come in for criticism. Phillips (2006a), for example, draws attention to the contradiction between countries such as Australia defending direct intervention in states which are presented as posing a threat to national security in the name of advancing democracy, whilst at the same time failing to adequately support a civil society response to women's personal security in the home.

As emphasized in the chapter on 'Men and Violence', the utility of focusing on explanations of domestic violence, particularly when this appears to promote individual and pathologising explanations has been questioned. Rather than looking for casual links, it appears to be more productive to view the naming and defining of domestic violence as a social process. This means that the naming and defining of violence will vary at both micro and macro levels relating to how both individuals and groups are positioned and how they position themselves.

It is also pertinent, at this stage, to review the findings from the World Health Organisation's *Multi-country Study on Women's Health and Domestic Violence Against Women*, produced in 2005 (World Health Organization [WHO], 2005). This study took as its starting point that violence against women by an intimate partner is a major contributor to the ill health of women. It recognized that previous research into domestic violence had not generally focused on non-western countries and that different indicators of violence had been used. This study collected evidence from 24,000 women from 15 sites in 10 countries with these sites representing diverse cultural settings. The countries represented were Bangladesh, Brazil, Ethiopia, Japan, Peru, Namibia, Samoa, Serbia and Montenegro, Thailand and the United Republic of Tanzania. This was primarily a population based survey to estimate the prevalence of violence against women across countries and cultures.

The findings showed that the proportion of women who had experienced physical or sexual violence or both from an intimate partner at some time in their lives ranged from 15 per cent to 71 per cent with most sites recording a prevalence level of between 29 per cent and 62 per cent. The greatest amount of violence was reported by women from rural and provincial settings in Bangladesh, Ethiopia, Peru and the United Republic of Tanzania. The lowest levels were recorded in Japan, but even here approximately 15 per cent of women reported experiencing physical or sexual violence or both at some time in their lives. Yokota (2006) notes that within Japan, emphasis continues to be placed on conservative family values, with the concept of 'gender equality' remaining a highly contested area. However, she emphasizes that there is a growing awareness of domestic violence and that the stories of survivors have been powerful in claiming public attention and bringing about political recognition.

When exploring connections between intimate partner violence and physical health, the WHO survey (2005) found that in the majority of the settings (with the exception of Japan, Samoa and urban areas within the United Republic of Tanzania) women who had experienced physical or sexual partner violence or both, were significantly more likely to report poor or very poor health compared with women who had never experienced partner violence. It was also found that recent experiences of ill health were associated with a lifetime's experience of violence, suggesting that the physical effects of violence may last long after the actual violence has ended or that cumulative violence has the most significant effect on health.

As noted in the chapters on men and violence (Chapter 3) and violence and aboriginal issues in Australia (Chapter 5), the factors affecting Indigenous women are complex. Statistics report high levels of violence against women in Indigenous communities in Australia (Taylor, Cheers, Weetra and Gentle, 2004). However, the difficulties involved in countering gendered power imbalances when communities, as well as individuals, experience persistent abuse and oppression, are considerable. As a result, it is vital that action is fully directed by Indigenous women to ensure that it achieves a positive effect for them in specific community settings. Humphreys (2007) comments that connections between violence against women and already existing health inequalities and social divisions constitutes a sensitive issue. She maintains that arguments which contend that violence against women cuts across classes and is not overtly condoned in any culture are too simplistic. Humphreys' suggests that a more complex discussion of this area is required and that full account needs to be taken of the compounding nature of social divisions, including increased barriers to help-seeking that may significantly increase isolation and entrapment.

It is also important to draw attention to mental health issues. The WHO (2005) study pertinently pointed out that across all settings and countries, women who had experienced physical or sexual violence or both by an intimate partner reported significantly higher levels of emotional distress than women who had not had these experiences. This is re-inforced by Humphreys (2007) who, in a review of research findings about the impact on women's mental health of gender based violence, found consistent negative connections. She points to heightened rates of depression, post-traumatic stress, attempted suicide and suicide, to maintain that the physical and mental health impact of violence against women is interconnected and substantial and constitutes a major public health problem. The WHO survey, mirroring the findings of Hearn (1996), also reported that women frequently consider emotionally abusive acts to be more devastating than physical violence. In the Survey these acts included being insulted or made to feel bad about oneself, being humiliated or belittled in front of others, being intimidated or scared on purpose and being threatened with harm. It was found across all of the countries included in the Survey that between 20 per cent and 75 per cent of women had experienced one or more of these acts mostly within the past twelve months. With regard to controlling behaviour by men towards women, this was seen to vary more significantly between countries with 21 per cent of women in Japan reporting such behaviour compared to almost 90 per cent in urban areas in the United Republic of Tanzania.

The WHO survey (2005) findings about mental health can also be associated with research currently being undertaken at the University of Sydney by Irwin and colleagues. They are discovering that women who have experienced domestic violence and who then become involved with mental health services are finding themselves subject to three main types of responses. The first is about 'silencing', with mental health service personnel not enquiring about or appearing to want to know about domestic violence. The second is linked to the first and refers to a mental health 'diagnosis' not taking domestic violence into account and the third shows how a mental health diagnosis can be used to discredit a woman's claims about domestic violence (Irwin, Waugh and Bonner, 2006). Although this research is in its early stages, it is being found that there is little communication between domestic violence services (which remain predominantly in the non-government sector) and mental health services, and that this lack of dialogue is causing further problems for women. A study by Humphreys and Thiara (2003) distinguishes between practices which could be located within a 'medical' model of mental health and those available in the non-medicalized voluntary sector. It was reported that medicalized services tended not to recognize the trauma that the women had experienced as a result of domestic violence and by focusing on women's health and the provision of medication rather than counselling rendered abusers invisible. They found the services and interventions which women did find helpful to be predominantly located within the voluntary sector. These included workers helping women name domestic violence, actively asking about abuse, attending to safety planning, responding to women's specialist needs and actively working with women to recover from abusive experiences.

At this juncture, it is useful to consider issues related to power, power imbalances and gendered divisions in more detail and here the work of Michel Foucault (1979, 1980, 1986) can be seen to have a useful application. As Fawcett (2000) points out, Foucault paid little attention to gender divisions, but importantly he did not view power as a thing or entity which some possess and others do not. He saw power as a productive force which circulates amongst people by means of 'taken-for-granted' social practices. His view of power is one where 'bottom-up' social practices are reinforced at the macro level and given added legitimacy, but he made it clear that macro practices do not add anything that is new or different but reinforce and consolidate what is already there. In relation to domestic violence, this highlights that gendered imbalances of power can become embedded in particular social practices making domestic violence more likely, but not inevitable between individuals in some communities in some contexts. This analysis is not presented to discount individual responsibility for perpetrators of domestic violence, but to make links between social forces and individual agency and to highlight the importance of challenging 'taken-for-granted' social practices both within and between countries.

In relation to issues associated with the perceived inevitability of domestic violence, it is also important to emphasize that although 'taken-for-granted' social, cultural and economic practices can be seen to, at times, make certain actions appear more acceptable to individuals or communities, challenge is always possible and the exercise of individual agency cannot be dismissed. To go back to the WHO survey (2005), a key finding was that although violence by a male intimate partner was widespread, there was considerable variation from country to country and from setting to setting within the same country. It was found that socio-demographic factors did not account for the differences between settings and the report highlights that 'the wide variation in prevalence rates signals that this violence is not inevitable'. It is important to note that an analysis that focuses on the circulation and use of power in everyday social practices does not necessarily claim that this process is equal. The circulation of power in social relations will occur differentially and as part of this process gendered power imbalances will foster intimate partner violence in some situations but not in others. Possible explanations of this and linkages to individual male narratives and how these are influenced by culturally, socially and economically orientated practices at micro and macro levels is clearly an area which warrants further exploration.

It is also pertinent to note, as part of this discussion, that contemporary social practices are located within a time period, which, whether referred to as embracing high modernity, late modernity, or post modernity, can be seen to have lost the all-pervasive, large-scale certainties of modernism. Progress is no longer regarded as inevitable or a 'good thing', scientific or social statements have ceased to be accepted as indisputable facts and the pronouncements of experts do not carry the weight they once did. However, in all of this, the need for certainty has not disappeared, but the large all-embracing certainties of modernism can be seen to have been translated into 'small certainties'. These 'small certainties' can be seen to operate in the rolling out of standardized professional practices which are unilaterally administered over an ever increasing number of areas of human need (Fawcett and Featherstone, 1998). 'Small certainties' are also promoted when some organizations, and an example is the Probation Service in England, decides that a particular therapeutic technique (and in this instance it is a form of cognitive behaviour therapy), represents '*the*' way to engage with diverse groupings of service users including those convicted of domestic violence offences. The imposition of these 'small certainties', by implication leads to the downgrading of process skills, of user led engagement and of interaction. Domestic violence, although clearly requiring an ethical imperative of zero tolerance, does not lend itself to the application of a standardized set of procedures that are seen to be universally applicable. It also cannot be viewed as a singular or straightforward issue.

At this point, it is also possible to relate this analysis to aspects of 'globalization'. The whole concept of globalization was initially driven by economic concerns and produced what appeared to be an all-embracing critique of welfare states, strongly regulated economies and high taxation systems. It continues to be presented as a driver for the increasing standardization of policies and practices in a wide range of areas. However, as commentators such as Fook (2002) have pointed out, changes which are regarded as world scale have different and contradictory expressions in different contexts. Looked at in this way, globalization, in one of its key manifestations, can perhaps be seen as an attempt, and it can be argued, a vain attempt, to counter increasing fragmentation and relativism and to re-impose the certainties of modernism into a world, which on every level, is becoming more multi-faceted and complex. With regard to domestic violence, this way of thinking has a tendency to gloss over power imbalances relating to gender, ethnic and social divisions and to present complex matters in unidimensional and straightforward terms.

A discussion of domestic violence in relation to intimate partner violence has to consider matters concerning domestic violence and children and the implications for the mother and here there are a number of points to make. In countries such as the UK and Australia, for example, domestic violence is increasingly being seen as a child welfare issue and mandatory reporting was extended in 1998 in Australia as part of the New South Wales Children and Young Persons (Care and Protection) Act. This places the requirement on agency personnel to report any instance of domestic violence where those concerned have children, to a child welfare agency. Mandatory reporting with regard to domestic violence was supported by many bodies including feminists, but its operation, as Ainsworth (2002) has pointed out, has been mixed. It has resulted in investigations focusing on the welfare of the child, but it has also tended to place more pressure on the mother, rather than serving as a mechanism for tackling male domestic violence. Ainsworth (2002) has also noted, in a comparative study focusing on Western Australia which does not have mandatory reporting, and New South Wales, which does, that mandatory reporting does not result in more cases of abuse being substantiated. He argues that it leads to the movement of resources away from services to children and families to services which concentrate on investigative and forensic activity.

Implications for human service professionals

At this point, it is helpful to turn again to the WHO survey (2005) in order to look at the responses of professionals and agencies to domestic violence. In the findings of this Survey, it is notable that a sizeable proportion of women did not tell anyone about the violence and/or abuse they were experiencing and those who did were more likely to tell family and friends than representatives from formal or statutory services. The low use of formal services can reflect in part the limited availability of services in many places. However, the study stresses, that even in countries relatively well supplied with resources, barriers such as fear, stigma and the threat of losing their children, prevented many women from seeking help. These factors provide a major challenge for all professionals working across different countries and in different contexts and questions relating to how social workers, health workers and members of statutory services can cut through cultural, social and political barriers to provide support which is viewed by the women concerned as appropriate and sensitive, have to be posed. Viewed as an individual, as a community and also as a costly and preventable public health issue, domestic violence clearly warrants a more coordinated, women-centred and supported response from professionals than has often, but, not always been the case. As has been highlighted, measures designed to help, such as mandatory reporting, have been double-edged and have tended to result in assessment and screening, rather than in the provision of resources that the women find useful. Mental health services can also ignore the impact that domestic violence has had on a woman's emotional wellbeing and at worst, a mental health diagnosis can serve to invalidate a woman's experience.

Moves to address these areas and to involve fathers who have been domestically violent in safety planning (Featherstone and Peckover, 2007), clearly signals a way forward. Similarly zero tolerance media campaigns in some countries have also made it clear that a range of violent behaviours by men towards women are unacceptable. Lih-Rong Wang (2006) points to the need for collaboration between service providers and argues that as social workers span a broad spectrum of human services agencies, they are well positioned to connect women with appropriate and sensitive services. Tsun On-Kee (2006) also highlights, as part of 'a frame of acknowledgements', the importance of professionals actively fostering inclusive approaches which acknowledge the resilience and skills of individuals and families. In responding to women who have experienced domestic violence there can be seen to be a clear role for professionals operating in a variety of areas to collaborate, to strengthen informal support networks and to work with women to generate the kind of support that they find helpful and useful. This is the current challenge and it is one which requires professional commitment, innovative and sensitive engagement with women as well as the allocation of adequate resources.

In conclusion, it is clear that domestic violence is differentially understood and responded to within and between countries. A consequence of this is that it frequently falls short of being seen as a human rights issue which requires government, community and professional responses. In this chapter it has been argued that domestic violence is intrinsically related to gendered power imbalances which have different manifestations in different social and cultural contexts. However, the view that violence is inevitable even when tacitly sanctioned by social, cultural and economic practices is challenged. It is emphasized in relation to domestic violence that although zero tolerance is an ethical imperative, the ways in which gendered power imbalances foster intimate partner violence in some contexts but not in others and the ways in which this can be explored without invoking traditional pathologizing explanations is an area which requires further investigation.

Chapter summary

Women and violence

- Domestic or intimate partner violence is a global issue which resonates throughout society.
- The manifestation of domestic violence in social relations reflects gendered power imbalances and social divisions.

(Continued)

(Continued)

- Domestic violence by women against men is gaining currency as a social issue. However, statistics continually show that the predominant form of domestic violence worldwide relates to violence towards women by men.
- Domestic or intimate partner violence can be viewed as constituting direct public violence or can be wider ranging incorporating emotional and sexual elements, threats, forms of humiliation and control.
- 'Abuse' can be defined as violence or can be seen as part of a continuum. It also creates associations with a wider range of settings including residential and resource centres.
- The naming and defining of domestic violence can be seen to be a social process which is linked to the position of the person or group undertaking the defining.
- The WHO (2005) study found significant connections between domestic violence and the physical and mental health of women who had experienced domestic violence in a worldwide context.
- The issues involving indigenous women are complex and it is vital that action is fully resourced by governments and that it is clearly directed by indigenous women to ensure a positive effect is achieved in specific community settings.
- 'Taken-for-granted' social, cultural and economic practices can make certain actions more acceptable to individuals or communities. However, as has been demonstrated worldwide, violence against women is not inevitable. Gendered power imbalances will foster intimate partner violence in some situations but not in others.
- Attempts to impose the certainties of modernism in a world which on every level is becoming more multi-faceted and complex glosses over power imbalances relating to gender, ethnic and social divisions and presents complex matters in straightforward and one-dimensional ways.
- Mandatory reporting in Australia can be seen to have placed more pressure on the mother, rather than serving as a mechanism for tackling male violence. It has also focused resources on investigative and forensic activity rather than on services to children and families.
- Human service professionals need to respond to women in ways which the women find helpful. Zero tolerance campaigns and involving fathers who have been domestically violent in safety planning have been found to be practices which obtain results.
- The ways in which gendered power imbalances foster intimate partner violence in some contexts but not in others and the ways in which this can be explored without invoking traditional pathologizing explanations, can be seen to be an area for further investigation.

3   Men and violence

Maurice Hanlon

Power and its manifestations in social relationships are key considerations in our understandings of men and masculinity. In this chapter men's violence towards others in the domestic sphere will be examined. The boundaries surrounding the meaning of violence continually shift and change to reflect cultural and social factors. Sanctioned violent enterprises or violent actions at both the state and the personal level can always be identified however. Reflected here we see huge differences in terms of income, class, formative experiences, gender cultures, and hegemonic aspirations. Although men dominate in the statistics concerning intimate partner violence, it has to be recognized that not all men are violent. This chapter will explore the theoretical perspectives which have been put forward to explain men's use of gendered violence. It will then examine key features which have emerged from the burgeoning literature dealing with men and masculinities over the past decade, before moving on to look at issues associated with violent men and fathering. This chapter, drawing from the literature will have a western focus, but will use perspectives and findings which have an international relevance.

However, before focusing on these areas, it is useful to refer to a summary of an interview carried out for a research project looking at the intergenerational experiences of British men. This interview will serve both as a point of reflection and as an illustrative case study when considering the material on men and violence.

David[1] was the eldest child in a large family. Money was often short and the family experienced a great deal of ill health and personal tragedy. His memories of his father are those of an aggressive man who was often involved in violent confrontations with other men. David recalls feeling constantly fearful of his father and being unable to talk to him. His dad was so tightly wound up that small things could promote immediate explosions. He also fuelled his anger by continually making connections between what was being said and previous areas of dispute and contention. As a result he was difficult to live with and David left home as soon as he could. However, given his father's background and his tragedies David feels he understood his father's particular way of 'getting through'.

David's background resulted in an initially not very coherent decision to 'do' masculinity differently. As a result he recounts that he further angered his father

---

1 Names have been changed to ensure confidentiality.

by not enthusiastically using the boxing gloves he bought him one Christmas, for not physically winning disputes with peers, and for trying to escape the harshness of the 'male' world by spending time with his mother in the kitchen and by trying to be like her.

Returning to the literature on violence, there have been many explanations and perspectives which have been put forward to explain men's use of violence and men's violence towards women. These have been critically appraised in the 'Women and Violence' chapter. However, it is worth looking at some of the more pervasive here. One explanation which has received considerable attention over the years maintains that violence in men is biologically determined. Accordingly, it is regarded as a natural instinct which men need to control with some men requiring more assistance than others in order to do this. This socio-biological explanation has now been widely critiqued in the men and masculinities literature (Pease, 2003; Connell, 2000), although it still continues to rear its head in political circles and in the media. Another popular frame of reference focuses on individual pathology and regards both perpetrators and victims as having developed a particular way of operating which both continues and escalates violent acts. This view is often associated with arguments drawn from social learning theory, where violent behaviour is seen as being learnt and then transmitted within and between generations. All of the above explanations fail to resonate with the experiences of David. They also ignore structural factors, power imbalances and the pervasive and insidious influence of dominant ideologies. All of these arguments, as highlighted in the previous chapter, personalize, individualize and privatize practices and actions which have wide ranging social consequences.

Other explanations emphasize social causational factors which focus on social and individual stressors precipitating violence at particular points. There are also interactive explanations which make connections between social structures and the ways in which these affect individual men, predisposing some to violent acts, to consider. This area has proved perhaps to be the most fertile area for exploration and has, tangentially in some cases, resulted in the far more nuanced and considered work by figures such as R.W. Connell, Jeff Hearn and Bob Pease. Aspects of these contributions will now be considered.

R.W. Connell's work is both extensive and comprehensive and complex arguments are made accessible by the use of pertinent examples from history and from research. It is difficult to isolate one aspect as all are interrelated, but Connell (1987, 2000, 2005) emphasizes the connection between gender and violence with regard to the institutionalized production of a narrowly defined hegemonic masculinity which influences and is in turn is influenced by, for example, the domination of men in the armed forces, in bodily contact sports and in road accident statistics. Masculinized management styles, which prioritize toughness, risk taking and ruthlessness about profits, with an associated insensitivity about the consequences of these actions for others, further reinforces this perspective. Connell (2000) dismisses arguments which flow from biological essentialist perspectives and says that testosterone levels, for example, far from being a clear cut source of dominance are more likely to be a consequence of social relations. Connell reinforces the message that although men have higher rates of violence than women, not all men are violent and argues that both the causes of and the answers to gendered violence have to be sought in social masculinities.

When looking at responses, Connell (2000) emphasizes that in multicultural societies there are likely to be multiple definitions of masculinity. Violent and aggressive masculinity is therefore seen as one form amongst others. This results in there being alternatives for anti-violence programmes to build on, to draw practical examples from and to publicize.

Connell (1987, 2000) acknowledges that the hierarchical way in which masculinity is organized can serve to police those who seek to distance themselves from hegemonic forms. Similarly the way in which violent masculinities are often institutionally supported and collectively defined, makes the promotion of alternatives an organizational issue. Connell (2000, 2005) emphasizes that the heterogeneous composition of masculinities contain tensions and contradictions which create space for change and maintains that the ongoing construction of masculinity can at various points give rise to both optimism, in that dominant hegemonic patterns are being eroded, and pessimism in that violent forms can be re-emphasized. Connell (2000) looks at masculinities in the context of globalization and highlights that a gender-formed strategy to move away from violence and towards peace has to be sophisticated about patterns of masculinity. It must also operate across a broad spectrum encompassing the development of children and young people, personal life, community life, cultural institutions, workplaces and labour, capital and commodity markets. Connell (2000; 2005) argues that the task is not to abolish gender but to reshape it, and to promote diversity by disconnecting, for example, courage from violence, steadfastness from prejudice, and ambition from exploitation.

Hearn's work is considerable and with regard to men and masculinities it encompasses a broad range of areas. He is critical of searching for casual explanations for men's violence towards women as this is often illusory. Hearn and Whitehead state:

> While it is quite possible to identify individual, family, cultural, economic, structural and other causes or explanations of violence, the search for a final cause may be futile. Explanations need to be treated with caution; they can be re-used to take moral and political responsibility from men individually and collectively, as 'excuses' or justifications for violence.
>
> (Hearn and Whitehead, 2006: 58)

An area which Hearn has focused on with Linda McKie (forthcoming) critically appraises both gendered policy and policy on gender by looking specifically at domestic violence. They draw attention to the wide ranging nature of violence against women, which includes the physical, sexual and the psychological as well as the economic. Drawing from national representative surveys and research they highlight that although strangers and acquaintances are responsible for the majority of crimes and assaults against men, women and children are more likely to be 'beaten, stalked, raped or killed' by intimate relatives or partners than by any other type of assailant. They contrast this with the policy arena where violence is portrayed as relating to identified perpetrators reinforcing the underlying assumption that violence in intimate relationships is atypical.

Hearn and McKie (forthcoming) examine three gendered processes of policy construction. These processes relate to: gendering the naming and defining of violence; gendering the locations and contexts of violence; and foregrounding the 'absent presence of men' in policy work and practices. With regard to the first area, Hearn and McKie draw attention to how the prominence given to any one perspective, definition or name reflects the shifting and contingent nature of power, domination and oppression. With regard to the second, they look at the ongoing segregation between the public and the private with governments, the state, agencies, families and individuals continuing to accept, reinforce and draw upon gendered inequities in the development and organization of policies and services. They also note how domestic violence policies often perpetuate such inequities, naming and defining the problem as the woman's problem which in turn is categorized as resolved once immediate safety issues have been dealt with. The third area concentrates on how it is only relatively recently that 'men' as individuals, groups or categories have been problematized and an assumed gender neutrality questioned.

Hearn and McKie (forthcoming) in an exploration of policy development at international levels, show that although sex discrimination legislation (despite some revisions) continues to gain mainstream momentum, active engagement with the ways in which gender shapes and reflects social relations is continually avoided. Such mainstreaming has also resulted, as Phillips emphasizes in her chapter, in the disbanding and sidelining of initiatives focusing specifically on gender and women. Hearn and McKie comment that in certain policy circles a specific focus on gender issues is seen to have served its purpose. They argue for the renewal of the concept of gender in policy work by increasing the engagement with theoretical pluralism and empirical research in order to make the impact of men and men's practices on the evidence base and on the processes of gender/policy analysis more explicit.

Pease (2003) takes a pro feminist stance and uses postmodern critical theory. He says that this perspective not only recognizes structural inequalities in men's lives, but also emphasizes the ways in which dominant discourses have shaped men's diverse subjectivities. This highlights the importance of locating men in the context of patriarchy and within the divisions of class, race, sexuality and other forms of social inequality, whilst at the same time exploring the ways in which patriarchal belief systems become embedded in men's psyches. As can be illustrated in the account by 'David', Pease draws from the work of Connell and Hearn to highlight that although systemic power imbalances generally work in men's favour, the structures of domination operate differentially, with factors such as 'race', sexuality, class, disability and age affecting the extent to which men can benefit from patriarchy. Differential access to avenues of masculine power can lead to marginalized groupings emphasizing particular male stereotypical characteristics which in turn have a particular impact on women in marginalized communities. Furthermore, hooks (1991) and others have drawn attention to the difficulties faced by women in marginalized communities where contact with organizations such as the police and welfare workers will result in further discrimination for the marginalized group as a whole. Pease (2003) also points to how systemic male dominance can deform men, resulting in emotional inexpressiveness and stress related conditions.

Drawing from Hearn and Pringle, Pease (2003) and Pease and Camilleri (2001) want to move away from a simple dichotomy of men portrayed as either perpetrators or victims to analysing men's practices in a range of areas. With regard to male violence and sexual coercion they stress the importance of challenging cultural values that promote aggression and the belief that male domination over women is a natural right. Drawing from Klein and colleagues (Klein, Campbell, Soler and Ghez, 1997), Pease emphasizes how cross-cultural research studies have shown the greater the level of gender inequality (bolstered by masculinity and femininity being seen as polar opposites) in a society, the higher the level of violence against women. He observes that intervention with perpetrators of violence often merely focuses on men's abuse of authority within the family rather than upon the nature and the constitution of the authority itself. He argues for analysing men's practices in key sites of sexual politics as a starting point for professional groups to work towards gender equality and to challenge the reproduction of patriarchal relations.

In a consideration of men and violence, it is important to look at the specific position of indigenous men. In Australia, Indigenous men have been subject to systemic discrimination and a devaluing of their contribution to the family and community since the first arrival of English settlers in 1770. Pearson (2000) has highlighted how violence has been clearly identified as an issue in Indigenous communities but points out that analysis and recommendations have been based on western perspectives and understandings. As a result, these have either proved unworkable or have further contributed to the colonization and oppression of Indigenous communities. Taylor and colleagues (2004) have drawn attention to how Indigenous communities have emphasized the significance of a well resourced holistic and community orientated response. They draw from the Canadian First Nations Aboriginal approach to highlight the: interlinkage of physical, spiritual, mental and emotional health; the impact of socio-economic problems such as poverty, unemployment and poor housing; the importance, but also the complexity of addressing gendered power imbalances when whole communities experience discrimination and oppression; and the need to locate the individual in the context of the family and the community.

Any discussion about men and violence has also to look at the issues surrounding violent men and fathering. Scourfield (2003), in the UK context, points to how women in child protection investigations are often left to manage men's behaviour and the consequences of such behaviour. Featherstone and Peckover (2007) emphasize that violent men continue to be regarded as perpetrators or offenders, but that their identities as fathers remain invisible. They highlight that this has serious consequences for the development of policies and practices which focus specifically on 'domestically violent fathers'. Featherstone (2004) significantly emphasizes that although there has been a considerable amount of work carried out with regard to men and masculinities in the last two decades, relatively little attention has been paid in this literature to men's practices as fathers. This contrasts with the considerable amount of work on fathers and fatherhood coming from the developmental psychology field which in turn has rarely engaged with the men and masculinities literature. This lack of dialogue between the two approaches can be seen to have resulted in issues relating to fatherhood, and gender, power and violence being insufficiently explored.

Fawcett, Featherstone and Goddard (2004) argue that in contemporary society, changing divisions of labour, changing work patterns, and changing aspirations on the part of women, in association with a weakening of other sources of attachment such as class, can result in children becoming the repository for feelings of stability which cannot be attained elsewhere. They assert that this causes children to become lost as people in their own right and to become ciphers for adult's feelings. This clearly can happen to mothers as well as fathers, but with regard to fathers can be associated with the current emphasis on 'men's rights' with regard to children which particularly comes to the fore in custody disputes.

As Featherstone and Peckover (2007) point out, researchers, such as Harne (2004), have found that many men who have been involved in violent relationships appeal to 'rights' discourses with regard to disputes about their children. Writers such as Eriksson and Hester (2001) suggest that conflicts over contact with children in situations where marriage is no longer a means of men controlling women can be seen as part of men's ongoing attempt to maintain control over women and children. Day Sclater and Yates (1999) however, take a different view and regard the 'men's rights' discourse around custody as an example of how some men publicly try to manage their masculinity in the contemporary world. They say that rights discourses can provide a means of reconstructing and translating private feelings of profound anxiety and vulnerability into a face-saving public exercise.

Following on from research with mothers who had left violent men, Radford and Hester (2006) argue that a key factor in determining visitation and contact arrangements between children and violent men is that mothers have to feel safe about such arrangements as it is in the child's best interests for further acrimony to be avoided. Williams, Boggess and Carter (2001) emphasize how violent men can use visitation rights to perpetrate control and continue harassment. They point to the different perspectives held by domestic violence and fatherhood movements and call for constructive collaboration. They also see healthy non-abusive behaviour by men who have battered, as a goal in the field of domestic violence. Featherstone (2004) sees fathers who have been domestically violent as being capable of change. She draws from her own research with a fathers' project and highlights how many young fathers talked of wanting 'to do it' differently from the way they had been fathered. She emphasizes that a number who were struggling 'to do it' differently spoke of a paternal legacy of hurt, anger, loss and lack of confidence which they lived with daily and also a lack of cultural back up or capital. She stresses that resulting tensions can lead to men expressing strong desires to negotiate respectfully with women around contact at one point and then hammering on their ex-partner's door at another when feeling alone and vulnerable.

Featherstone and Peckover (2007) and Scourfield (2003) maintain that as part of offering better intervention to women and children, men as fathers need to be fully engaged. They make it clear that it is not a question of moving funding away from services for women and children to finance programmes for violent men, but that safety planning for women and children must include work with men. In this, their argument is underpinned by the ethical position which recognizes the imperative of not condoning violence, but which engages with the men and masculinities literature. Accordingly, they argue for account to be taken of the complexities of men's individual life histories, how hegemonic masculinity becomes interwoven with local gender orders, and how this plays out under current conditions of gender instability.

The interview summary provided at the outset gives an example, at the individual level, of how one man, 'David', sought to make sense of his father's behaviour. He clearly found this unacceptable and has chosen to 'do' masculinity differently, yet this is combined with an understanding of the structural factors and particular pressures which influenced his father's behaviour.

Implications for human service professionals

Men's violence to women can be wide ranging and human service professionals need to be aware of the controlling and insidious nature of violence which contains within it aspects of abuse and oppression at physical, emotional and economic levels. The safety of women and children has to be paramount, whilst at the same time violent men's capacity to change has to be constructively addressed. As has been emphasized, this is not about mothers and fathers, men and women competing for the few services or support lines available, but recognizing that all, in different ways, have specific needs and claims. Men's violence towards women has to be tackled at a social level with violent practices and the underpinning rationale being consistently challenged. However, as has been highlighted in all the chapters in this book, there is a clear role for service providers to play. This includes interrogating taken-for-granted gendered claims, whilst at the same time actively listening to what men and women, fathers and mothers, have to say about their experiences and the pressures and expectations placed upon them. It is about identifying and building on strengths as well as challenging unacceptable practices and it is about exploring the differential impact of patriarchy by men on men.

Chapter summary

Men and violence

- Central to an understanding of men and masculinity is the notion of power.
- The work of Connell emphasizes how in multicultural societies there are multiple definitions of masculinity which provide alternatives for anti-violence programmes to draw on.
- Hearn and McKie maintain that in relation to international policy development although sex discrimination legislation, despite some switchbacks, continues to gain mainstream momentum, active engagement with the ways in which gender shapes and reflects social relations is continually avoided.
- Pease argues for men's practices to be analysed in key sites of sexual politics as a starting point for professional groups to work towards gender equality and to challenge the reproduction of patriarchal relations.
- Indigenous men have been subject to systemic discrimination and devaluation. When whole communities experience compounded disadvantage and stigmatization, ways forward need to highlight the interlinkage of physical, spiritual and emotional matters and the grinding impact of poverty, unemployment and poor housing.
- With regard to fathers who have been domestically violent, Featherstone and Scourfield maintain that as part of offering better intervention to women and children, men as fathers need to be fully engaged.
- With regard to human service professionals, the safety of women and children has to be paramount whilst at the same time violent men's capacity to change has to be fully addressed.

4   Trapped within poverty and violence

Deborah Hart

> At the heart of any consideration of poverty lies the issue of what is needed to live 'a decent life' and more fundamentally, what it is to be human.[1]

> The court outcome today gives me strength to believe that I deserve to be treated better and it helps me to … start to believe that I am as valuable as other people.[2]

The above quotes were selected to open a chapter on 'poverty and violence' because they illustrate the humanity that is sometimes hidden behind scholarly accounts of these distressing life experiences. The first quote refers to an emerging understanding of poverty that goes beyond a purely technical assessment of income requirements towards a focus on quality of life measures. The second quote reminds us that people have a capacity to exercise strategic agency and resilience when confronted with the material and emotional consequences of poverty and violence but this requires a social, economic and legal climate that is conducive to sustainable recovery and healing.

As other chapters in this book demonstrate, violence, abuse and oppression are committed across the entire economic spectrum and in all social groups as defined by age, race, ethnicity and sexual orientation. However, research provides evidence of a clear link between poverty and violence within relationships and communities. Broadly speaking, this link encompasses the oppressive power dynamics that can result from relationships of emotional and material dependence as well as the restricted options available to people who lack adequate material resources to shape their own lives and futures.

This chapter will focus on challenges faced by people who live in poverty to escape from relationships that are dominated by violence, abuse and oppression. The discussion begins with a broad consideration of connections between poverty

---

1 Uniting Care Australia Submission (number 13) to the 2004 Australian Government Senate Community Affairs References Committee Inquiry into Poverty and Financial Hardship.
2 Quote from Ms Fee Fen Njoo following a charge of assault against her former partner (*Sydney Morning Herald Weekend Edition*, 20–21 January 2007).

and violence in a global context. It then moves on to provide an explanatory framework for conceptualizing multidimensional interactions between poverty and violence as a first step in the process of evaluating policy and practice interventions in relation to their capacity to promote safety and wellbeing for people, regardless of their economic circumstances.

A number of specific questions will be addressed in this chapter. First, in what ways might the experience of violence be different for people living in poverty? Second, how do current and emerging social and economic policies and practices maintain oppressive relationships of dependence? Turning this question around, what social and economic policies and practices promote opportunities to escape violence, abuse and oppression? Finally, why is it important for human service professionals to be aware of the complex interconnections between poverty and violence? This chapter will explore these broad questions within a global context while providing specific illustrations within the Australian policy and practice environment.

Framing the links between poverty and violence: global considerations

At the most elementary level, it can be argued that the toleration of absolute poverty across the world is itself a perverse form of systemic violence. On a global scale, there are obscene disparities in material wealth and prosperity between 'overdeveloped countries' (Choules, 2006) and the 40 per cent of the world's population surviving on less than US \$2 per day (United Nations Development Programme, 2005: 4). Despite significant economic growth in many countries of the world, absolute poverty and inequality continues to grow within impoverished nations and within certain groups in more affluent societies (World Bank, 2005).

It is clear that women and children experience the material and emotional impact of poverty and relationship violence acutely (Sen, 1999; Lister, 2004; Phillips, 2006b). This is due to a broad range of factors including: women's traditional caring commitments and consequent economic dependence; the unequal distribution of income and consumption within families; gender divisions within global labour markets, and income disparities between men and women that appear to be increasing with the deregulation of economies (Stilwell, 2006) and industrial relations systems (Peetz, 2007).

A recent United Nations Children's Fund (UNICEF) study into the material wellbeing of children across Organization for Economic Cooperation and Development (OECD) countries shows that some of the most affluent nations in the world, including the United States of America (USA), the United Kingdom (UK) and Australia are performing badly across a range of quality of life measures for children (UNICEF, 2007a). The wellbeing of children is intimately connected with issues of gender equity across the globe. In the words of Kofi Annan, the former Secretary-General of the United Nations (UN), 'When women are healthy, educated and free to take the opportunities life affords them, children thrive and countries flourish, reaping a double dividend for women and children' (UNICEF, 2007b: vi).

Violence against women and children is committed across all nations, regardless of socio-economic conditions. However, extreme poverty appears to be the direct cause of some specific forms of violence against women and girls in impoverished regions of the world. Watts and Zimmerman (2002) describe a rapidly growing worldwide industry in the trafficking of women and girls for forced labour and sexual exploitation. They refer to studies that show that this illicit trade in women and girls is driven by armed conflict, global and internal displacement, economic and social inequities, combined with a demand for low-wage labour and sex work (Watts and Zimmerman, 2002.). Amnesty International highlights the particular vulnerability to violence, abuse and oppression of refugee women, and women displaced in their own country due to gender-based persecution and violation (Amnesty International, 2004).

Given the magnitude of material deprivation experienced by the majority of the world's population, what possible hope could people who live in the midst of absolute and degrading poverty have of escaping violence, abuse and oppression? This question goes to the heart of what the development economist Amartya Sen calls the 'agency aspect of the individual': the capabilities a person has to 'act and bring about change in order to achieve the substantive freedoms he or she enjoys to lead the kind of life he or she has reason to value' (Sen, 1999: 87). Sen conceptualizes poverty as the deprivation of these basic capabilities to live a decent life, rather than merely as lowness of income.

To Sen, freedom from poverty, violence, abuse and oppression is predicated on sustained international initiatives and institutional reforms that promote opportunities for individuals and communities to exercise strategic agency. These reforms include, among other things: expanding the access of poor nations to the markets of richer countries; urgent attention to global arrangements for curbing an arms trade that is sustained by wealthy nations, and making patent laws and incentive systems fairer to allow access to life-saving medical treatments for the poorest communities (Sen, 2006). Human service professionals in developing countries and increasingly in affluent nations are confronted on a daily basis with the casualties of poverty and violence in their work with people who have been violated through global displacement, global market forces and emerging punitive welfare reform measures.

The experience of violence, abuse and oppression for people living in poverty

It was argued in the previous section that poverty and violence have similar trajectories in that both life experiences limit capabilities, prevent choice and inhibit access to safety. Elspeth McInnes conceptualizes the multidimensional and multidirectional interconnections between poverty and violence through her statement that 'the impact of poverty essentially compounds the impact of violence, while violence both creates and extends poverty' (McInnes, 2004a: 1).

The remainder of this chapter will explore the connections between poverty and relationship violence, beginning with a critical appraisal of research findings that demonstrate a clear connection between violence and poverty. The chapter will conclude with an examination of the implications of these research findings for policy and practice frameworks.

It is important to stress from the outset that a majority of people who are poor do not violate others and do not directly experience material violence in their lives. On the other hand, many people who are affluent violate others, sometimes in the pursuit of wealth, or become the target of various forms of violence themselves. This chapter begins from an assumption that people at every level of income have the capacity to make choices about committing violence or escaping from violence, but these choices can be constrained by the material conditions under which people live and the policy and practice climate that circumscribes options.

As is the case with any complex issue within the field of human services, the arguments and analyses presented here are subject to debate and challenge. Debate begins from the moment any attempt is made to conceptualize, measure and analyse specific aspects of poverty or relationship violence. Attempts to artic-ulate links between poverty and violence introduce further layers of complexity and grounds for contestation. The challenge when mounting any argument about links between poverty and violence is the difficulty of teasing apart causal relationships.

What is the research evidence for connections between poverty and violence within relationships and communities, and why is this question important? Human service professionals see evidence on a daily basis of the over-representation of people on low incomes seeking assistance because of relationship violence. However, efforts to draw attention to links between poverty and relationship violence can arouse a reflexive response that warns of the potential to single out and further stigmatize people who already experience multiple forms of social and economic disadvantage (Tregeagle, 1990; Hood, 2001; Evans, 2005).

While this is a legitimate concern, avoiding a critical examination of contested links between poverty and violence may have the effect of reinforcing a popularly held belief that violence only happens to an 'underclass' of poverty stricken people and communities in nations and suburbs far away. This construction of 'the poor' as 'Other' through language and images (Lister, 2004: 100) focuses attention on perceived individual deficits rather than the environments that con-tribute to and sustain social disadvantage. Consequently, unrealistic expectations are placed on individuals who are most at risk of poverty and relationship violence to rehabilitate themselves within these poorly resourced environments (Hood, 1998). This individualizing discourse is a feature of emerging welfare reform measures in Australia (Australian Council of Social Services [ACOSS], 2005); the United Kingdom (Dean, 2003) and the United States (Reid and Tom, 2006), and in recent domestic violence policy initiatives in Australia (Evans, 2005; Murray, 2005; Watson, 2001); the UK (Ferguson, 2003) and the USA (Scott, London and Myers, 2002).

Following McInnes (2004a), this brief review of the literature will focus on studies of relationship violence that explore the proposition that poverty causes or compounds violence, before moving on to examine the ways in which violence creates and extends poverty. It is clear that the former proposition is more contested than the latter but it is important for human service professionals to be aware of a broad range of explanations for the links between poverty and violence in order to work towards best practice in the field (Evans, 2005).

Explaining the links: poverty causes or compounds violence

The proposition that poverty causes or compounds relationship violence is highly contested amongst those feminist scholars and practitioners who argue that relationship violence is caused by patriarchal power dynamics. This line of argument suggests that any effort to theorize alternative contributing factors provides an excuse for violent and oppressive behaviour.

One argument that runs counter to this proposition is that men who are disempowered and humiliated by poverty express their lack of power through violence towards others, most often women and children. Returning to developing nations for just a moment, Amartya Sen, in his analysis of armed conflict across extensive regions of the world, argues that we have to understand more clearly how poverty, deprivation and neglect, and the humiliations associated with asymmetry of power, relate over long periods to a propensity for violence (Sen, 2006). According to Sen, the sense that the world is divided between 'haves and have-nots' contributes to the 'cultivation of discontent', opening up the possibilities of recruitment in the cause of what is often seen as 'retaliatory violence' (Sen, 2006: 146).

James Gilligan poses a related argument in his statement that people who are relatively poor in affluent societies are more likely to be disrespected and treated as less than human and the feelings arising from such treatment make violence more of an option (Gilligan, 1996 cited in Evans, 2005: 40). Evans also cites a study by Garbarino (1999) that concludes that the effects of poverty and other social inequalities allow boys to develop an 'impaired inner world' that enables a perception that violence towards women and children is acceptable (Evans, 2005: 40).

Barbara Miller takes a similar position in her analysis of intracultural aggression and violence within some indigenous communities in Australia. Miller argues that the socialization of Aboriginal children, in particular boys, in a colonized discriminatory environment can interact with frustration and conflict to cause aggression and violence (Miller, 1990, cited in Memmott, Stacy, Chambers and Keys, 2001). In an earlier study of interpersonal violence in one particular Indigenous Australian community, Jill Atkinson found that Indigenous women expressed concern and feelings of helplessness, 'knowing their sons will grow up and beat their wives and show no respect for women' (Atkinson, 1990: 10).

A study by Malcoe, Duran and Montgomery in the USA led to similar findings in relation to Native American women who live under severely depressed socio-economic conditions (Malcoe *et al.*, 2004). Indigenous people in both nations have been subjected to colonization and concomitant abuse and oppression, with severe disruption to traditional gender roles and family relationships. These and other studies conclude that high rates of intimate partner violence in Indigenous communities can be attributed to the substantially higher poverty rates that have been caused by a long history of systemic racial violence.

An emerging body of research from the USA offers support for economic and structural explanations for differential prevalence rates of relationship violence. Tolman and Raphael (2000) review a significant number of empirical research studies on the incidence rates of reported domestic violence in the USA and conclude that rates of domestic violence are considerably higher for women who are poor than for women in the general population. Not only is the prevalence rate higher for women in receipt of low incomes, there is also evidence that the severity of violence women sustain is associated with receipt of welfare support and therefore poverty (Marshall and Honeycutt, 1999 cited in Tolman and Raphael, 2000). Lyon (2000) reports on research in the USA that establishes a clear connection between poverty, domestic violence and frequent periods of unemployment and welfare receipt, with unemployment often being caused by ongoing workplace harassment of women by abusive partners.

While there have been relatively few empirical studies conducted on this topic in Australia, the conclusions reached in these studies have consistently shown significantly higher incidence rates of reported domestic violence occurring among the most relatively disadvantaged social groups (for example, Chung, Kennedy, O'Brien and Wendt, 2000; Di Bartolo, 2001). Mary Hood reports on a study conducted in South Australian hospitals of admissions for children who have been abused. Her results provide evidence of an overwhelming connection between child abuse reports and poverty, unemployment and family disruption (Hood, 1998). Hood focuses on child sexual abuse and argues that in her sample, someone other than the mostly female parent is more often confirmed as having abused the child. Hood proposes that not having access to enough money leads many sole parents to experience emotional stress as well as poor housing, limited access to transport, and child care that is below the standard required by parents to ensure their child's safety and wellbeing. In these situations, according to Hood, sole parents and their children are at risk of predatory behaviour by perpetrators of sexual violence who seek out children and families with needs for financial help (Hood, 1998). A similar dynamic exists on a global scale with thriving child sex tourism markets in many impoverished nations (Seabrook, 2000).

Tony Vinson (2007) has assembled a substantial body of data on the distribution of social disadvantage throughout Australia that enables us to see the ways in which disadvantageous conditions are inter-correlated. Vinson provides evidence of a convergence of indicators in the lives of people who reside in specific geographical localities that sheds light on the foundations of disadvantage. Vinson's study demonstrates that localities with markedly high rankings on forms of disadvantage such as low income, family breakdown, early school leaving, disability, sickness, long-term unemployment and criminal convictions are areas in which child maltreatment is also more likely to come to notice (Vinson, 2007).

Tony Vinson does not set out to use these findings to further stigmatize disadvantaged people and communities but instead highlights indicators of cumulative social disadvantage that appear to be conceptually related. According to Vinson, this information 'has the capacity to provide a pragmatic administrative tool that can [be used by government administrations] to either focus restorative endeavours or anticipate and help prevent a local area's slide towards entrenched disadvantage' (Vinson, 2007: 98). It is essential for human service professionals to be aware of this complex and multidimensional connection between poverty and child maltreatment, and other forms of relationship violence, in order to provide effective and supportive interventions at a local level.

These and many other research studies demonstrate a clear correlation between poverty and violence in relationships and communities. While such studies provide a useful starting point for thinking about risk factors for relationship violence, they do not necessarily provide a framework for conceptualizing the factors that cause violence, abuse and oppression for people living in poverty. As other chapters in this book show, the dynamics of relationship violence are about power and control. Given that relationship violence occurs across the whole social and economic spectrum, how can we understand the higher prevalence and severity of relationship violence for poor individuals and communities?

Paul Memmott and his research colleagues focus on the prevalence of violence in Indigenous Australian communities and propose a framework for understanding the causes of relationship violence that may have relevance to an analysis of links between poverty and violence in a broader sense (Memmott *et al.*, 2001). This framework appears to offer a useful starting point for understanding the multidimensional and relational causes of violence for disadvantaged individuals and communities. Memmott and colleagues begin from an assumption that the primary explanation for violence is the oppressive exercise of power and control but they argue that three levels of causation mediate this dynamic: underlying factors, situational factors and precipitating factors (Memmott *et al.*, 2001).

Underlying factors are described as 'deep historical circumstances' that make particular communities vulnerable to violent behaviour (Memmott *et al.*, 2001: 18). In relation to Indigenous people, these factors relate to consequences of the structural violence of race relations over five or more generations (Memmott, 1991; also see Behrendt, 2003). For non-Indigenous Australians, underlying factors are historical and systemic forces that relegate certain individuals and communities to 'the lowest rung' (Peel, 2003). These factors relate to broad structures of inequality that characterize modern capitalism and exclude people from economic prosperity based on social divisions such as class, gender, race and disability (Stilwell, 2006). An understanding of underlying factors is important for a holistic approach to tackling relationship violence that stems from multiple systemic causes, including poverty and social exclusion.

Memmott and his colleagues describe situational factors as experiences that exacerbate violence in combination with direct causes. These factors may include loss of employment, family breakdown, financial problems and prevailing attitude towards violence in society and within communities (Memmott *et al.*, 2001).

These situational factors contribute to incidents of violence but are not direct causes of violence. Precipitating factors are defined as a type of social event that triggers a violent episode by a perpetrator, such as the perpetrator being intoxicated, a partner not having a meal prepared in time or quarrelling children (Memmott *et al.*, 2001). The intersection of these various factors can, according to Memmott and colleagues, result in highly possessive and exclusive interpersonal relationships that increase the vulnerability to violence for impoverished individuals and communities (Memmott *et al.*, 2001).

In summary, it is proposed that entrenched social disadvantage and social exclusion compounds interpersonal tensions and trigger events that can ignite violence within oppressive relationships of dependence. However, regardless of the very real systemic factors that contribute to violence, abuse and oppression within relationships and communities, it is clear that women and children continue to suffer the material and emotional consequences of that systemic violence and this can compound or extend their own experience of poverty.

Explaining the links: relationship violence causes or extends poverty

While the view that poverty causes or compounds violence remains contested, there can be little doubt that violence causes or extends poverty, particularly for people who are in any form of relationship of dependence with those who have violated them. Such relationships of dependence may include those between: people with a disability and their carer(s); between children and parents; adolescents leaving parental care or out of home care (see Mendes and Moslehuddin, 2004), and between people who are dependent on others to secure legal citizenship status. The difficult decision about whether to leave an oppressive relationship of dependence may rest on a person's perception of their capacity to enjoy a reasonable quality of life once the decision is made to seek emotional and material independence. This in turn rests on the social and economic policy context that influences access to social provisions during the process of making decisions about the future.

The remainder of this section will focus on the experience of relationship violence for women in Australia who are in oppressive relationships of dependence with a partner. While the remainder of this chapter will focus to some extent on women and children leaving violent relationships, the decision-making and safety planning process can apply to people in all social groups who are subject to violence, abuse and oppression. It will be argued that violence causes or extends poverty for diverse groups of people who are in the process of making decisions about escaping violence because they generally carry the economic and emotional costs of that violence (Laing, 2001; McInnes, 2004a).

Regardless of socio-economic status, relationship violence is likely to cause health and/or emotional impairments, including physical injury, anxiety and depression and post-traumatic stress disorder (Fraser, 2003; Schechter, 2000; Taft, 2003). Additional costs associated with these health and emotional impairments can create financial hardship in themselves and may also lead to barriers to sustainable, long-term financial security and protection from continuing abuse.

Violent relationships are much more likely than non-violent relationships to break down (McInnes, 2004a; Rawsthorne, 2006) and people at risk of violence may have to escape their homes and communities to protect themselves. When people are forced to escape violence at short notice, there is little opportunity to plan for economic security and those who are forced to leave situations of relationship violence face personal and social disruption that often results in financial hardship (Senate Community Affairs Reference Committee [SCARC], 2004).

People escaping relationship violence and abuse, regardless of their income and employment status, incur additional financial costs, including: housing and relocation costs; replacement costs for furniture and other possessions; additional consumption related costs associated with lost household economies of scale; increased legal costs to protect themselves and their children; loss of wages, and additional child care expenses (Access Economics, 2004).

According to Davies, Lyon and Monti-Catania (1998), women who experience abusive relationship are forced to analyse risks of staying in violent situations in relation to the costs of leaving that relationship. This is referred to as a process of 'active and ongoing safety planning' (Davies *et al.*, 1998: 73) and reflects a woman's capacity to understand her situation and to provide for the safety of herself and her children (Davies *et al.*, 1998). This is a complex decision-making process that is made more challenging when current or potential financial hardship restricts options for escaping abusive relationships. It could be argued that this safety planning process applies to the broad and diverse group of people who are forced to escape violence, abuse and oppression.

The capacity of people to plan for safety depends on the existence of social and economic policies and practices that promote opportunities to escape situations of violence, abuse and oppression. While there is a raft of formal policies that seek to address violence in most affluent countries, people need to feel confident that these policies and programmes will not place them and any children at risk of long-term poverty and social disadvantage should they decide to leave a violent relationship.

Broadly speaking, safety depends on the existence of supportive policies and programmes that promote sustained emotional and material independence and wellbeing. These policies must take account of the diversity and complexity of people's lives and of the work–life balance people escaping violent situations must have in order to achieve a decent life for themselves and their children. Specifically, policies and programmes that support transition to independence can include: assistance to obtain suitable accommodation; access to ongoing and sustainable employment; access to flexible education and training resources; economic support during the transition to financial independence and appropriate child care where necessary. Crucially, people who are actively considering escaping violence also need access to human service professionals who can act as advocates for them as they negotiate new and confusing systems of social assistance.

Safe and stable housing is a critical issue for people escaping violence. In the situation of women and children escaping violence, the best possible scenario is to remain in the family home if it is safe to do so and for the violent partner to leave or to be removed. In these situations, women and children remain close to familiar supports and children are not forced at a time of crisis to change schools and move away from friends and valued extra-curricular activities (Edwards, 2004). In many situations this option is not viable so women and children are required to seek temporary accommodation, either with family and friends or in many instances, in crisis accommodation. Demand for crisis accommodation for all groups of people escaping violence in Australia, for example, far outstrips availability and while women's refuges provide a supportive environment for vulnerable women and children, they are generally over-crowded and can only provide temporary respite from the need for secure housing. There are even fewer options for appropriate crisis accommodation for women without children or women with sons over the age of twelve.

The transition from crisis accommodation to stable and affordable independent housing is becoming increasingly difficult for people on low incomes as housing affordability becomes a critical issue and as government investment in social housing in Australia and the United Kingdom is declining. As a result of the decline in public housing stock, eligibility for subsidized housing is increasingly restricted to those people who experience multiple and complex problems that include, but go beyond poverty. A legacy of poor public housing estate planning, in addition to concentrating residents with multiple and complex life problems in social housing is exacerbating entrenched poverty and social exclusion.

The experience of relationship violence has been identified as a barrier to sustainable employment, both directly and indirectly (Butterworth, 2003). A direct barrier to employment arises when an abusive partner interferes with a woman in her workplace or hinders her efforts to improve her skills or education (Costello, Chung and Carson, 2005; Swanberg, Logan and Macke, 2005; Tolman and Raphael, 2000). Indirect barriers to employment are incurred when people are forced to move away from their home, family and friends to escape violence.

Costello and colleagues (2005) highlight the importance of employment as a pathway out of poverty for women and their dependent children affected by domestic violence. Costello and her colleagues draw on empirical studies that conclude that additional benefits from ongoing paid employment include: social reconnections; development of self-esteem, confidence and self-worth and a sense of efficacy in the world and acceptance by society (Costello *et al.*, 2005: 256). Employment service providers and human service professionals need to be aware of the connections between domestic violence and employment in order to provide effective assistance to women who are seeking independence and financial stability.

People who rely on welfare payments to support themselves experience hardship due to low rates of payment, increasingly stringent activity requirements and penalties, and inadequate government funding for employment assistance and other forms of social support such as child care services (ACOSS, 2005; SCARC, 2004). While relative poverty is a fact of life for people who depend on social security payments as their main form of income, the overall poverty rate for low-income families, including sole parents has been reduced over the past twenty years due to income support and tax measures (ACOSS, 2005). The Australian Child Support Scheme provides a mechanism for ensuring non-resident parents contribute financially to the support of their children and research has shown that this approach to redistributing income has lifted many children out of poverty, relative to families in the past. Child care subsidies for people on income support payments and low incomes assist increasing numbers of women to secure additional income from employment and therefore to find a level of financial independence.

While acknowledging government progress in mediating factors that cause child poverty, the Australian Council of Social Service identifies troubling trends in relation to family poverty arising out of emerging welfare reform measures and labour market changes in Australia (ACOSS, 2005). These trends are particularly concerning for people who are sole parents attempting to balance work and child care commitments. The Australian Government *Welfare to Work* policy draws from those in the United States and the United Kingdom and moves a significant number of sole parent families and people with disabilities onto lower income support payment rates and imposes new requirements on sole parents to seek paid employment if they wish to remain eligible for income support payments to raise children.

While there is limited empirical research available to assess the impact of this new policy on people escaping relationship violence, there is a significant amount of literature coming out of the United States that shows that welfare reform policies are having a detrimental impact on women who have escaped domestic violence (eg. Long, 2001; Murphy, 1997; Scott *et al.*, 2002; Tolman and Raphael, 2000). Broadly speaking, US workfare policies have significantly reduced the number of sole parent families receiving income support payments but advocates for 'battered women' who are no longer eligible for welfare support argue that a proportion of these women have become vulnerable to returning to abusive relationships of dependence or forming new abusive relationships in order to survive financially.

Implications for human service professionals

Human service professionals in every field of practice are working at different levels of intervention with people who confront poverty and violence on a daily basis. These interactions take place within a context of institutional and managerial reform that places increasing emphasis on cost containment and risk management at the expense of the dignity and welfare of service users. Many human service workplaces are implementing standardized assessment tools to inform complex decision-making processes, while under-resourcing and tight deadlines can lead to rushed decisions that do not take full account of the complex lives services users lead. This can provide particular challenges for human service professionals when working with people who are in the process of making safety-planning decisions.

It is imperative for human service professionals to remain aware of the complex intersections between poverty and violence in order to avoid the imposition of yet another layer of abuse – 'institutional abuse' – on people who are at some point in the process of escaping violence. Abuse constructed at the institutional level can result from unintended but damaging racial and gender prejudice (Forbat, 2004); stereotyping of impoverished people (Peel, 2003); inadequate funding and coordination for essential programmes; lack of time for critical reflection and professional development, and inadequate support for human service workers who confront crisis and trauma on a regular basis. Whatever the cause of institutional abuse, the outcome can be critical for people living in poverty who are weighing up their options for escaping violence, abuse and oppression.

In conclusion, it can be said that poverty and violence feature in the lives of far too many people across the globe. Regardless of where we are born, we all hope for a decent life that rewards our efforts to contribute to our families and communities. The experience of poverty and relationship violence deprives people of the opportunity to apply their various capacities and to exercise strategic agency to shape their lives in ways that they value. This chapter has argued that poverty itself is a form of unnecessary systemic violence. Many people across the world are trapped in poverty due to economic, legal and social policies that are beyond their control to influence. Many others are trapped within relationships of individual, community and systemic violence because they lack the material resources to escape.

This chapter provides a snapshot of a range of explanations for the ways in which poverty can cause and compound various forms of interpersonal violence at a global and a local level. It was suggested that there continues to be debate and contestation about the causal connections between poverty and violence but a common factor in all these analyses is a motivation to better understand the mechanisms that assist people and communities to escape the material and emotional consequences of these unnecessary and distressing life experiences.

It has been demonstrated that for social and economic policies to be effective in allowing people to escape violence, abuse and oppression, they need to be informed by an understanding of the complexity and diversity of people's lives. It has also been argued that human service professionals have key support and advocacy roles to play in their work with people during their transition from oppressive relationships of dependence to a life of safety. Human service professionals are in the better position to provide effective interventions when they understand the complex and multidimensional relationships between poverty and violence.

Chapter summary

Trapped within poverty and violence

- Research evidence demonstrates a clear link between poverty and violence within relationships and communities.
- The link between poverty and violence encompasses the oppressive power dynamics that can result from relationships of dependence as well as the restricted options available to people living in poverty to escape from abusive relationships.
- There is an active debate about the causal relationship between poverty and violence, with some people arguing that the indignity of living in poverty causes some men to take out their frustrations on women and children.
- It is widely accepted that violence causes and extends the experience of poverty for women and children.
- It has been suggested that while violence is caused by the oppressive exercise of power and control, there are underlying, situational and precipitating factors related to poverty that mediate this power dynamic.
- People who experience abusive relationships have the capacity to exercise resilience and strategic agency to plan for their safety but this requires a social and economic climate that is conducive to taking action.

5 Towards healing

Recognizing the trauma surrounding Aboriginal family violence

Karen Menzies and Lorna McNamara

Aboriginal communities in Australia experience violence – sexual assault, family violence and child abuse – at rates far in excess of the wider community (AIHW [Australian Institute of Health and Welfare], Al-Yaman, Van Doeland and Wallis, 2006). This violence is primarily perpetrated on Aboriginal Australians by other Aboriginal people (Fitzgerald and Weatherburn, 2002). It is argued in this chapter that in order to understand this violence and abuse and to develop appropriate responses, it is imperative to locate the current violence within the context of the historical and traumatic experiences endured by Aboriginal people as a result of unjust and oppressive state policies and practices. This will be illustrated using the example of child welfare policies and practices in the Australian state of New South Wales (NSW), examining both their implementation over time and their traumatic legacies from colonization to the present day.

A structural-feminist trauma framework is used to explore the impact of Aboriginal child welfare practices and as a vehicle for developing culturally appropriate responses. While it is recognized that feminism as a movement has had particular limitations when applied to the experience of Aboriginal people (Moreton-Robinson, 2000), this framework provides the basis for analysis of trauma at the levels of the individual, the family and community. Importantly, it places responsibility for the trauma in the hands of the dominant culture and structures. This framework also offers guidance in the healing of individuals and communities, sustained by broader political change.

> To hold traumatic reality in consciousness requires a social context that affirms and protects the victim and that joins victim and witness in a common alliance. For the individual victim, this social context is created by relationships with friends, lovers and family. For the larger society, the social context is created by political movements that give voice to the disempowered.
>
> (Herman, 1992: 9)

Implications for human service professionals of working from these contextualized understandings of the complexities of violence and abuse in Aboriginal communities will be demonstrated through a discussion of some of the activities of the Education Centre Against Violence (ECAV), an agency within the NSW Health Department. ECAV provides an example of a mainstream organization engaged in a collaborative partnership with Aboriginal leaders active in addressing family violence, sexual assault and child abuse across NSW. Through the partnership, an understanding of the historical context and its legacies on the current environment in Aboriginal communities has evolved, enhancing the development of training and community-based programmes.

The history of Aboriginal child welfare in NSW

Examining the history of child welfare policy has two purposes. The first is to provide a context for understanding the present. The chronicle of evolving policy and practice reveals that although the thinking about Aboriginal people changed over time, there was and is a continuing pattern of institutionalized racism. Secondly, this analysis of history helps to show the cumulative impact of government policies on Aboriginal children and families: not just on one individual but on multiple generations of parents and children; not just on one family but on whole communities. Each policy has left its own indelible mark on Aboriginal people. When the health and wellbeing of Aboriginal Australians is measured against internationally accepted indicators, it is clear that these policies have had profound effects (Standing Committee on Aboriginal and Torres Strait Islander Health and Statistical Information Management Committee, 2006).

According to a research report by the NSW Law Reform Commission, Aboriginal child welfare can be grouped into four discreet periods characterized by the introduction of legislation, policies and practices governing Aboriginal children (NSW Law Reform Commission, 1997: 13). These periods are briefly summarized in turn.

Colonial period 1788–1883

> McMillan gave the instruction to surround the camp … The Kurnai attempted to escape. Some raced into the scrub only to be met by stockmen who gunned them down. Others jumped into the waterhole. McMillan and his men positioned themselves around the waterhole and, as fast as they put their heads up for breath, they were shot until the water was red with blood.
>
> (Elder, 1998: 99)

It is crucial to our understanding of Aboriginal history and culture to recognize that the colonization of Australia by Europeans in 1788 was achieved by force. This marked the beginning of the dispossession of land and the erosion of culture and identity for Aboriginal people. Aboriginal people had well-established social laws, rituals, customs and spiritual beliefs that were intrinsically linked to the land (Atkinson, 2002). The imposition of European ways and Christian beliefs began at this time. For example, an institution was established in the settlement in 1814 with the purpose of educating Aboriginal children away from the influence of their families (NSW Law Reform Commission, 1997: 13). This period marks the first phase of practices involving the forcible separation of Aboriginal children from their families.

Protectionist policies 1883–1937

> Angus McMillan led massacre posses against the Kurnai in the 1840s and by the 1890s was the local Protector of Aborigines.
>
> (Elder, 1998: 98)

In 1883 the Aborigines Protection Board was established. Its aims were clear:

> The Board reasoned that if the Aboriginal population described by some as a 'wild race of half castes' was growing, then it would somehow have to be diminished. If the children were to be de-socialised as Aborigines and re-socialised as Whites, they would somehow have to be removed from their parents.
>
> (Dr Peter Read Submission, cited in Human
> Rights and Equal Opportunity Commission, 1997: 33)

Initially the Aborigines Protection Board relied on inducement and coercion of parents to remove children (NSW Law Reform Commission, 1997: 17). In 1909, the passing of the Aborigines Protection Act in New South Wales gave the Aborigines Protection Board far greater power to remove children. Parental consent or a court order was no longer required. Children could be removed from their families if it was considered to be in the interest of the child's physical or moral welfare. In some instances, the reason recorded for the removal of a child by the Aborigines Protection Board was simply 'for being Aboriginal' (NSW Law Reform Commission, 1997: 18).

In 1915 the Aborigines Protection Amending Act gave complete power to the Aborigines Protection Board to remove Aboriginal children from their families and put them into training homes. The girls were trained for domestic service and the boys for farm labour. The homes were harsh, regimented and loveless environments where children were indoctrinated to despise their race, their culture, their families and, by implication, themselves (Swan and Raphael, 1995).

Assimilationist policies 1937–69

> At the age of four, I was taken away from my family and placed in Sister Kate's home – Western Australia where I was kept as a ward of the state until I was eighteen years old. I was forbidden to see my family or know of their whereabouts ... The Protector of Aborigines and the Child Welfare Department in their 'Almighty Wisdom' said that we would have a better life and future bought up as whitefellas away from our parents in a good

religious environment. All they contributed to our upbringing and future was an unrepairable scar of loneliness, mistrust, hatred and bitterness.

(Millicent, Human Rights and Equal Opportunity
Commission, 1997: 115)

In the late 1930s Australia officially adopted the policy of 'assimilation'. In New South Wales this happened in 1937. Assimilation officially became the philosophical underpinning of the laws governing Aboriginal people. The stated intention of the policy of assimilation was to make all persons of Aboriginal descent live as members of a single Australian community, to attain a similar manner and standard of living, to enjoy the same rights and privileges, to accept the same responsibilities, and be influenced by the same hopes and loyalties as other Australians (NSW Law Reform Commission, 1997: 18) – notwithstanding that Aboriginal Australians were not given the right to vote until the 1960s and were not counted in the census as Australian citizens until the Referendum in 1967.

It was not until the NSW Act was amended in 1940 that children were required to be brought before the Children's Court under the provisions of the Child Welfare Act (1939). Children could be removed if they were found to be 'neglected' and 'uncontrollable' and if they were subjected to 'improper' or 'incompetent' parenting. Too often these terms of reference were exaggerated or fabricated for the courts. Aboriginal children could be and were removed on the grounds of 'neglect' if they were in the care of a relative (Burns, Burns, and Menzies, 1999: 161).

In the 1950s excessive overcrowding in Homes for Aboriginal children and prohibitive costs led to Aboriginal children being placed with non-Aboriginal foster families. Assimilation continued in the homes of foster parents. According to Commissioner Wooten (1989) who conducted the Royal Commission into Black Deaths in Custody, these assimilation policies and programmes were tantamount to genocide in terms of the United Nations' definition under the Convention on the Prevention and Punishment of the Crime of Genocide (NSW Law Reform Commission, 1997: 22).

1969 to the present

This time I was raped, bashed and slashed with a razor blade on both my arms and legs because I would not stop struggling and screaming. The farmer and one of his workers raped me several times. I wanted to die, I wanted my mother to take me home where I would be safe and wanted ... When they returned me to the home I once again went to the Matron. I got a belting with a wet ironing cord, my mouth washed out with soap and put in a cottage by myself away from everyone so I couldn't talk to the other girls. They constantly told me that I was bad and a disgrace and if anyone knew it would bring shame to Sister Kate's Home ... I ate rat poison to try and kill myself but became sick and vomited. This meant another belting.

(Millicent, Human Rights and Equal Opportunity
Commission, 1997: 115)

The Child Welfare Act (1939) had a much more detrimental effect on Aboriginal than on non-Aboriginal children (Tatz, 1991). Terms like 'neglect' were still applied to Aboriginal children found in the care of relatives by non-Aboriginal workers who had a poor understanding of the notion of the extended family in Aboriginal culture. Workers refused to place some children with relatives on the grounds that housing was 'over-crowded'.

Although recent child welfare legislation such as the NSW Children and Young Persons Care and Protection Act (1998) has attempted to redress past practices, for example, by including sections on Aboriginal participation, the rate of Aboriginal children and young people on child protection orders continues to be higher than the rate for other Australian children (Australian Institute of Health and Welfare, 2006).

The next section of this chapter will look at the impact of these policies on Aboriginal families and communities.

The impacts of child welfare policies of separation

Consequences of childhood separations

Both the immediate and the long-term traumatic impacts of separation of children from primary caregivers are well documented in the psychological literature. This literature emphasizes that the quality of adult social relationships is profoundly affected by an infant's first experiences (Wolkind and Rutter, 1984). In particular, the loss of a mother in childhood may lead a person to become excessively prone to developing psychiatric symptoms, especially when current personal relationships are problematic (Bowlby, 1988: 174). Discordant or disruptive family relationships in early life and a marked lack of parental affection are both associated with a substantially increased likelihood of both emotional disturbance and personality disorders in adult life (Wolkind and Rutter, 1984). Disrupted parenting in infancy or early childhood leaves the person less secure and more vulnerable to adolescent and adult psychological and emotional disturbances.

These impacts are compounded for Aboriginal children forcibly removed from their families because they were alienated from their Aboriginal roots yet were not accepted by 'white' society, thus becoming alienated from both cultures (Lynch, 2001). This ultimately renders Aboriginal people vulnerable to what has been termed 'acculturative stress' (Williams and Berry cited in Ward, 1997). 'Acculturative stress' is defined as the 'stresses inherent in simultaneously striving to preserve one's cultural heritage, negotiating one's relationship with the dominant culture and having to deal with the racism and discrimination which one might encounter on a regular basis' (Williams and Berry cited in Ward, 1997).

The effect of forcible separation policies and practices was that Aboriginal children were denied the basic social structure of a family. They were denied the fundamental universal human right – the right to parental love, their family, other familial relationships and knowledge of their cultural identity – because their cultural heritage was viewed as 'undesirable'. Aldgate describes this process as 'breaking prematurely the lifeline of the developing child' (1988: 36).

The loss Aboriginal children experienced in being torn from family and culture, and the loss of families and communities that saw generation after generation of children removed from their arms, has resulted in a burden of grief both profound and disabling. The trauma of loss and grief is ubiquitous across Aboriginal communities (Atkinson, 2002; Swan and Raphael, 1995).

The experiences of Aboriginal children living under assimilation policies, suffering abrupt and often permanent forcible separation from parents and families, can be compared to the experiences of Jewish children caught up in the Holocaust (Beresford and Omaji, 1999: 194). Such experiences are associated with profound alterations in the self and in relationships and inevitably result in the questioning of basic tenets of faith: 'When we lose a loved one, we lose a part of ourselves. When so much of the self is removed at once, a disorientation ensues, an emotional paralysis follows' (Hass cited in Beresford and Omaji, 1999: 195).

Childhood abuses

> In 1935 … the manager of Kinchela Boys Home [was advised] 'to give up taking intoxicating liquor entirely' and 'that on no account must he tie a boy up to a fence or tree, or anything else of that nature, to inflict punishment on him, that such instruments as lengths of hosepipe or a stockwhip must not be used in chastising a boy, that no dietary punishments shall be inflicted on any inmate in the Home'.
>
> (NSW Aboriginal Protection Board cited in Elder, 1998: 218)

While the trauma of removal embedded itself in the memory of many of its childhood victims, their subsequent experiences in institutions and foster homes added new layers of emotional distress (Beresford and Omaji, 1999: 197). These included both the effects of institutionalization – living in an institution or substitute family where the child was not nurtured, loved or cared for by warm and supportive parents, and horrific experiences of physical and sexual abuse.

The effects of institutionalization erode personal emotional development and damage the individual's sense of self-worth. The same factors also have an impact on health, housing and employment prospects. Psychological and emotional torment leaves many people less able to develop social and survival skills. This may result in a decreased ability to operate successfully in the world and impair or limit educational achievements and ultimately restrict employment prospects.

There are many well recognized psychological impacts of sexual abuse and physical abuse in childhood. They include inability to trust, verbal and physical aggression, confusion of sex with love, difficulty with emotional regulation and aversion to sex and intimacy. When the child is blamed or is not believed about the sexual abuse, other psychological impacts can be added. These include guilt, shame, lowered self-esteem and a sense of being different from others (Wolfe, Gentile, and Wolfe, 1989: 195). 'The impact amounts to a variant of post-traumatic stress disorder, involving sleep disturbances, irritability, fears, anxiety and depression' (Brayden, Deitrich-MacLean, Dietrich, Sherrod, and Altemeier, 1995: 1254–5). Commonly for survivors of child sexual abuse the inner conflict of betrayal continues into adulthood and ultimately affects their ability to maintain intimate relationships with partners and offspring.

The documented effects of forced separation, institutionalization and child abuse on Aboriginal Australians

In 1995 the Human Rights and Equal Opportunity Commission conducted a major inquiry into the historical practice of forcibly removing Aboriginal children. The *National Inquiry into the Forcible Separation of Aboriginal and Torres Strait Islander Children from their Families*, commonly known as the 'Stolen Generations' Inquiry, produced the *Bringing Them Home* Report (Human Rights and Equal Opportunity Commission, 1997). The Inquiry found that the predominant aim of Aboriginal child separations was 'the absorption or assimilation of the children into the wider, non-Aboriginal community so that their unique cultural values and ethnic identities would disappear, giving way to models of Western culture' (Human Rights and Equal Opportunity Commission, 1997: 232). For example,

> When me and my little family stood there – my husband and me and my two little children – and all my family was there, there wasn't a word we could say to each other. All the years you wanted to ask this and ask that, there was no way we could ever regain that. It was like somebody came and stabbed me with a knife. I couldn't communicate with my family because I had no way of communicating with them any longer. Once that language was taken away, we lost a part of our very soul. It meant our culture was gone, our family was gone, everything that was dear to us was gone.
>
> (Fiona's story, Human Rights and Equal Opportunity
> Commission, 1997: 111–12)

Many Aboriginal people recounted stories of physical brutality and sexual abuse by welfare officials or other 'carers'. The testimonies in the report detail such commonalities in experiences of abuse and neglect at the hands of those charged with the care of children that they cannot be explained as isolated incidents from one or two institutions or one particular foster or adoptive family. Common experiences revealed in evidence and submissions presented to the Inquiry included the following: lack of stability; physical and cultural separation; poor living conditions; sexual and physical abuse; absence of any meaningful bonds; poor education; and exploitation through work. Despite the emphasis on religious and 'moral' training, sexual abuse of the children was common, both within the institutions and where girls were sent out to domestic service. For example, Archbishop Donaldson, visiting Barambah settlement, noted that of the girls sent out to service 'over 90 per cent come back pregnant to a white man' (Burns *et al.*, 1999: 164).

For many Aboriginal people, the trauma of their forcible separation generates ongoing feelings of insecurity, feelings of hopelessness, helplessness, marginalization, and discrimination over a lifetime. One witness to the Inquiry illustrates the persistence of vulnerability during her life by stating:

> 'I now understand why I find it so very, very hard to leave my home, to find a job, to be a part of what is out there. I have panic attacks when I have to go anywhere I don't know well and feel safe. Fear consumes me at times and I have to plan my life carefully so that I can lead as "normal" an existence as possible. I blame welfare for this. What I needed to do was to be with my family and my mother, but that opportunity was denied me.' Confidential submission 483, South Australia: woman fostered at 18 months in the 1960s.
> (Human Rights and Equal Opportunity Commission, 1997: 169)

The deliberate and systematic attempt to destroy Aboriginal Australians culturally and emotionally was (and continues to be) felt and internalized by individuals and communities today. According to Muriel Bamblett, Chairperson of the Secretariat of National Aboriginal and Islander Child Care (SNAICC): 'It is important not to dismiss these losses as simply belonging to the past but acknowledge how important these losses are for Aboriginal people today' (Bamblett, 2004: 29).

Understanding trauma – a place to start

The *Bringing Them Home* Report concluded that trauma became an inescapable end result for Aboriginal children. Trauma is an overwhelming experience of fear and helplessness. Traumatic events can involve threats to life or bodily integrity, or a close personal encounter with violence or death. Traumatic events that are experienced directly include, but are not limited to, military combat, violent personal assaults, being taken hostage, terrorist attack, natural disasters and incarceration in a concentration camp (American Psychiatric Association, 1994: 424). It is important to note that even when the threat has gone, or the event is long over, traumatized people relive the event as though it were continually recurring in the present.

Only relatively recently, and largely due to the work of feminist psychiatrist Judith Herman, have child abuse and abuse of women within their intimate relationships been acknowledged as also constituting traumatic events. Herman's feminist critique of traumatology is clearly relevant as she states that: 'the study of psychological trauma must constantly contend with the tendency to discredit the victim or to render her invisible' (1992: 8). Herman highlights the powerful role played by society's response, not only in the restitution of the trauma, but in defining and accepting it as a traumatic event in the first place. Too often, however, the most traumatized and vulnerable members in society are denied even minimal social support and community assistance, especially rape victims, child abuse victims, and many oppressed Aboriginal peoples around the world (Figley, 1985).

To try to make sense of the breakdown of social structures in Aboriginal communities without an understanding of the historical context, is to perpetuate further violence upon an indigenous society, already brought to its knees by state sanctioned violence, oppression and neglect.

Intergenerational trauma and collective trauma

Psychiatric definitions of trauma such as the delineation of symptoms comprising post-traumatic stress disorder (American Psychiatric Association, 1994) cannot adequately convey the nature and scope of the trauma that Australian Aboriginal people and other colonized indigenous peoples have suffered, nor its ongoing expression, for example, in high rates of violence, self-harm and drug and alcohol abuse (Atkinson, 2002; Burstow, 2003). Writers such as Judy Atkinson (2002) have argued that the concepts of 'transgenerational trauma' and 'collective trauma' more accurately convey the compounding effects of trauma for Aboriginal communities. Originally applied to understanding survivors of the Holocaust and their families (Perlesz, 1999), the concept of transgenerational trauma conveys the insidious and unconscious transmission of the effects of the trauma from one generation to the next.

Every single Aboriginal person is directly affected by the forcible separation laws, practices and policies, and continues to feel the effects of trauma and loss. It is unlikely that any other Australian today would have great-grandparents, grandparents, and parents who were starved, murdered, forced off traditional lands, imprisoned and/or stolen from their mothers. Because of this unique experience of Aboriginal Australians, the concept of collective trauma (Erikson, 1976, 1994) conveys an even more comprehensive understanding of how trauma experiences of forcible separation impact on Aboriginal people. According to Erikson the impact of collective trauma is defined as a 'blow to the basic tissues of social life that damages the bonds attaching people together and impairs the prevailing sense of community' (1994: 233). Collective trauma, by its very definition, poses a direct assault on the continuity and integrity of the cultural system. In a similar vein, Eisenbruch (1991: 674) uses the term 'cultural bereavement' to describe the experience of the uprooted person or group resulting from loss of social structures, cultural values and self-identity. As a result, there is an enormous 'load' of trauma and grief borne by Aboriginal people across generations that is expressed as violence, injury, poor parenting, unresolved grief, depression and mental illness (Human Rights and Equal Opportunity Commission, 1997).

It should be acknowledged that some Aboriginal people have not had the opportunity to develop this analysis or use this information to frame their own experience.

Understanding violence in Aboriginal communities in context

The concepts of transgenerational trauma and collective trauma provide the context for understanding violence in Aboriginal communities. For many Aboriginal communities, violence has become endemic. This violence is complex and occurs between immediate and extended family members and across generations. The violence once perpetrated against them by settlers and Government policies and practices is now played out between community members and within families. For example, based on reports to police, Aboriginal people in NSW are significantly over-represented as both victims of crime and as offenders compared with the population overall (Fitzgerald and Weatherburn, 2002). Aboriginal people are between 2.7 times and 5.2 times more likely than residents of NSW as a whole to become victims of violent crime (Fitzgerald and Weatherburn, 2002).

This over-representation as victims of violent crime is most extreme for Aboriginal women who experience sexual assault at a rate of 159.3 per 100,000 (compared to a rate of 57.3 for NSW women as a whole) and domestic-related assault at a rate of 1774.6 per 100,000 (compared to a rate of 337.5 for NSW women as a whole) (Fitzgerald and Weatherburn, 2002). Given that crimes of personal violence in general are under-reported to police because of factors such as fear and shame and given the history of poor relationships between Aboriginal people and the police, this data, though shocking, is a conservative measure of the extent of the violence experienced by Aboriginal people.

Rates of child sexual assault are also much higher for Aboriginal children (84.8 against 31.6 per 100,000) (Fitzgerald and Weatherburn, 2002). The Aboriginal Child Sexual Assault Taskforce identified that child sexual assault in Aboriginal communities 'is a grossly underreported crime'. It also noted that: 'When asked if they could think of a family in their community that had not been affected by child sexual assault, no Aboriginal person who took part in the consultations could' (Aboriginal Child Sexual Assault Taskforce, 2006: 60).

The state of Aboriginal communities today has a 200-year genesis. Entrenched racism at institutional and societal levels sustains and maintains a tolerance to violence that would be unacceptable should it occur in the broader community. Despite years of oppression, neglect and abuse, many Aboriginal women and men are speaking out about the violence in their communities in an attempt to protect their children and rebuild Aboriginal society. The courage to speak out, however, can bring its own dilemmas. Without a thorough understanding of the trauma to which Aboriginal people have been subjected, there is a risk of compounding pejorative stereotypes already existing at the service delivery level and in the broader community. As Marcia Ella Duncan, Chairperson of the Aboriginal Child Sexual Assault Taskforce (ACSAT) notes:

> This report contains data and research that describes a stark picture of intergenerational abuse and social disadvantage. ACSAT has continuously considered the potential impact of this on the Aboriginal community's perception

of ourselves, and how others perceive us ... ACSAT has tried to present its findings in the same spirit it found among communities. That is, in a way that is open and generous, acknowledging the issues are serious and complex, while at the same time as adamantly stating that it wants the abuse to stop, healing to begin and a better future for our children.

(Aboriginal Child Sexual Assault Taskforce, 2006: 2)

Recognizing the links between trauma and violence does not diminish the need to shape responses soundly located in understandings of accountability and responsibility. These are central to addressing the pain and suffering brought about by family violence and child abuse. As Aboriginal people gather strength to address family violence, sexual assault and child abuse within their communities, human services must also dramatically shift their focus to ensure genuine partnerships are developed. Resolution of these complex issues is only possible through community participation. Services must understand the context surrounding Aboriginal family violence, if this process is to succeed.

Implications for human service professionals

Understanding trauma begins with rediscovering history. In the same way that healing from traumatic experiences such as sexual assault and domestic and family violence requires that society hear the survivor and acknowledge the harm inflicted, there is an urgent need to hear and see the survivors of assimilation. Yet as Henry Reynolds (2000) notes, when it comes to the traumatic experiences of Aboriginal people, there is 'The Great Australian Silence' and 'the cult of forgetfulness' (Reynolds, 2000: 91–2).

It is salutary for human services professionals to recognize that interventions by health, welfare and legal agencies can compound the trauma experienced by Aboriginal communities by failing to recognize and address the underlying issue of trauma and by practices that enforce Aboriginal people's sense of powerlessness (Atkinson, 2002). Health and welfare services that are based on traditional models of practice which do not make the link between forcible separation and the trauma-related behaviours evident in Aboriginal communities today will fail to meet the needs of Aboriginal people and will perpetuate the tendency to blame the victim, rather than recognizing that:

> the problems of alcoholism, unemployment, [violence] and high mortality rates are not, as white society has argued for nearly two hundred years, endemic to Aboriginal people as a race. They are problems which are a result of a universal human response to dispossession and despair.
>
> (Elder, 1998: 255)

The compounding of trauma and trauma symptomotology is evident in populations denied recognition of their ordeal. This is notable in the experiences of Vietnam Veterans who struggled for decades to have their symptoms recognized as war related. Once these experiences were understood as a traumatic response, service provision was transformed to address their needs. Services that work with officially recognized traumatized individuals such as Vietnam Veterans, use relevant trauma literature (Herman, 1992: 70). Similar trauma-related behaviours of Vietnam Veterans can be seen in Aboriginal people who experienced forcible separation. The identification and validation of the experience is necessary not only for individuals but also to shape and guide the interventions.

In order to develop culturally appropriate policies and practices, partnerships between Aboriginal communities and non-Aboriginal organizations need to be equal. This means that the principle of self-determination must be incorporated. This principle holds a key to the health and wellbeing of Aboriginal communities. It allows Aboriginal people to make decisions about healing the past, the security to live in the present and the right to plan their own destinies. There are various examples where Aboriginal communities are acting in an advisory capacity in relation to matters directly affecting them. Aboriginal involvement at every stage of the process and at all levels must be a fundamental principle. The following section of the chapter provides an example of the operation of this principle in a partnership between Aboriginal people and a mainstream organization in the development of training and community education addressing violence and abuse for Aboriginal communities.

The Education Centre Against Violence (NSW Health) – an example of working together with Aboriginal people

In recognition of the impact of trauma on health, the Education Centre Against Violence (ECAV) has provided training and resources to health service providers in the areas of sexual assault, domestic and Aboriginal/family violence and child abuse for over twenty years. From its inception, there has been a commitment to Aboriginal training, with an understanding that Aboriginal educators were a vital link in understanding the needs of Aboriginal people and communities. In 1997, ECAV increased its role with Aboriginal communities when it entered into a partnership with the Centre for Aboriginal Health (NSW Health), to develop and deliver a competency-based qualification specifically addressing Aboriginal family violence. The course was to be developed in line with the Aboriginal Family Health Strategy, and targeted Aboriginal Family Health workers employed across NSW.

Historically, ECAV operated primarily from a feminist philosophy, which placed patriarchy at the centre of understandings of gendered violence. This philosophical base provided a sound platform for the development of service responses focused on sexual assault and domestic violence. As the Centre expanded its reach to include the mental health and disability sectors, as well as providing responses to Aboriginal and culturally and linguistically diverse communities, it was necessary for these understandings to be extended and refined. The inclusion of child protection and same-sex violence to the Centre's brief further accelerated this transition.

As the partnership with the Centre for Aboriginal Health developed, ECAV began in earnest to explore the competing philosophical and theoretical constructs of violence in order to effectively engage with the issues confronting Aboriginal communities and workers. The overriding philosophical framework which now supports models of training developed and delivered by ECAV relies on the complex interplay between understandings of the historical, cultural, legal, social, psychological, biological, political and personal contexts of those who have experienced interpersonal violence and the power relations affecting their lives and their access to services. A gender analysis is an integral part of this understanding, but it is addressed within these contexts and not in isolation.

The funding provided by the Centre for Aboriginal Health initially funded one Aboriginal and one non-Aboriginal temporary educator positions. In 2002 the positions were made permanent and in line with ECAV's increasing awareness of issues for Aboriginal workers, both positions were designated as Aboriginal. At this time ECAV was asked by the Aboriginal educator team to further extend the organization's role to actively include Aboriginal representation in decision-making affecting Aboriginal programmes, training and the Aboriginal workforce – that is, to incorporate the principle of self-determination into the partnership.

In 2003, following extensive consultations and discussions, the Aboriginal Community Matters Advisory Group (ACMAG) was formed. The aims of the group were to: provide advice and direction to ECAV on service delivery models, programmes and training; to provide a pathway into and a community voice for programme development within ECAV; to provide support to the ECAV Aboriginal workforce; and to provide advice and policy consultation to NSW Health and other government departments on sexual assault, family violence and child abuse. The impact of this consultative process was immediate and profound. With a strong and knowledgeable Aboriginal advisory group supporting the decision-making processes within ECAV, the Aboriginal educator team was able to more confidently and effectively engage Aboriginal communities and organizations around issues of Aboriginal family violence.

The training team for most Aboriginal training programmes up until this time included one Aboriginal and one non-Aboriginal educator. This model was regarded as best practice in the delivery of programmes to Aboriginal and non-Aboriginal workers providing services to Aboriginal communities, as it exemplified the notions underpinning reconciliation. Training programmes offered through this model were very successful, with the additional benefit that each educator had the opportunity to take significant learning from the other. However, with both educator positions being designated as Aboriginal, and with an increasing number of programmes being delivered to Aboriginal workers and community members only, ACMAG suggested that the model for Aboriginal specific training be shifted where possible, to an all Aboriginal training team.

It became evident from participant feedback that by delivering some workshops to Aboriginal workers and community members only and by prioritizing an all Aboriginal training team specifically for this training, there were significant, unanticipated benefits. First, there was an increase in the amount of participant feedback indicating appreciation of having training delivered by an Aboriginal training team. For example:

> Was inspired and encouraged seeing two Aboriginal trainers doing what they do. It has encouraged and empowered us to believe that we can go on to do bigger and better things with our lives.
>
>> (Participants, Wallaga Lake Child Protection Training, 2007)

> First training I have been to with Aboriginal trainers and Aboriginal class and can't believe how much more I have relaxed and learnt. The comparison is huge.
>
>> (Participant, Forster Child Sexual Assault Training, 2007)

Comments such as these suggest that the Aboriginal educators present powerful role models who are taking a strong stand against family violence and child abuse. For some participants who have had limited access to education, it enables them to visualize the possibility that they might with time, emulate the trainers and become confident, educated role models for their communities. Feedback of this type led ECAV and the ACMAG to surmise that perhaps workshops where there was a mixed training team, implied inadvertently to some that the knowledge base primarily rested with the non-Aboriginal educator. An all Aboriginal training team challenges this notion.

Second, there was an increased capacity to address the often hidden and deeply held shame of some participants, of not having had an adequate education. Fears of being 'dumb', struggles with reading and writing and expression through written activities, were more readily discussed and addressed by Aboriginal educators. This was particularly significant in the Aboriginal Family Health qualification course. Many participants have provided feedback to the effect that, if the course had been open to non-Aboriginal workers, they would have been unwilling to express and therefore address these fears. For example:

> I was so scared to come to this training as I did not know what to expect and what level of education the rest of the room would have. I left school in year eight and feel very inadequate academically. After getting to know both the Aboriginal trainers and the other entire Aboriginal participants I then realized that they all have similar stories. I now feel excited and comfortable to come and better my skills and academic levels in a safe and non-judgmental environment with other powerful strong Aboriginal women. Can't wait till next training when we all come together again.
>
>> (Participant, Aboriginal Family Health qualification course, 2006)

Another component of ECAV's partnership with the Centre for Aboriginal Health was the delivery of training to mainstream, non-Aboriginal workers. This training both explained the role of the Aboriginal Family Health Strategy (1992) and also placed Aboriginal family violence in context. Over the years 2004–06

ECAV developed and piloted a number of programmes, each building and improving on the last. The final evolution of the course, *Competent Responses to Aboriginal Sexual and Family Violence*, was delivered in 2006 and is now in considerable demand from departments across government.

This course outlines the cumulative impact of generations of violence and abuse on Aboriginal communities. It provides a clear demonstration of how the impact of trauma has been interpreted as failures within individuals and Aboriginal people as a race, marking them as lazy, less intelligent and biologically prone to alcoholism. The course encourages workers to reflect on the stereotypes and entrenched racism inherent in policies and practices that promulgate these myths and challenges workers to take into account the broader social and political context in order to provide respectful, culturally appropriate and meaningful interventions. The course has been well received with strong participant feedback that is exemplified by these comments:

> You have both inspired me to make changes in my work practice as well as personally.
>
> (Evaluation, 2003)

> [My most significant learning was] the generational expense of these issues, the multi layered impact on Aboriginal culture.
>
> (Evaluation, 2007)

In conclusion it has been argued in this chapter that a major factor in the exacerbation of trauma is the lack of acknowledgement of the harm inflicted, at both the personal and political levels. Once it is publicly recognized that a person has been harmed, the community must take action to assign responsibility for the harm and to repair the injury, a process that is essential to promoting healing and reconnection (Herman, 1992). In the situation of collective trauma experienced by Australia's Aboriginal people, acknowledgement of the history and ongoing traumatic effects of assimilation policies and practices is crucial if effective action is to be taken to address the legacies of violence and abuse, so evident today. This is the sentiment expressed by Alex Boraine, Vice Chair of the South African Truth and Reconciliation Commission, at the Aboriginal Reconciliation Convention (1997):

> Turning the page
> It's right to turn the page.
> But first you have to read it.
> You have to understand it.
> You first have to acknowledge it
> And then you turn the page.
>
> (Boraine, 1997)

Chapter summary

**Towards healing: recognizing the trauma
surrounding Aboriginal family violence**

- Aboriginal communities in Australia experience violence at rates far in excess of the wider community. This violence can only be understood within the context of the historical and traumatic experiences endured by Aboriginal people as a result of unjust and oppressive state policies and practices, exemplified by child welfare policies that resulted in the forcible removal of generations of Aboriginal children from their families.
- The psychological trauma inflicted on the individuals through forced separation from family, community and culture, compounded by the effects of living in cold and loveless institutions and foster homes and the abuse and neglect inflicted by 'carers', has been documented in the *Bringing Them Home* Report of the Human Rights and Equal Opportunity Commission. Every Aboriginal person has been affected by these policies.
- The concept of psychological trauma provides a starting point for understanding the impact of these policies and practices, but where whole communities and generations are affected, the concept of transgenerational and collective trauma better explains the extent of the suffering of all Aboriginal people and its current expression through violence, self-harm, mental illness and substance abuse.
- Aboriginal people are speaking out about the violence in their communities in an attempt to protect their children and rebuild Aboriginal society. This includes the recognition that responses must be located in understandings of accountability and responsibility.
- Human service providers must dramatically shift their focus by developing service responses that acknowledge the harm that has been inflicted and that develop genuine partnerships incorporating the principle of Aboriginal self-determination. The partnership between the Education Centre Against Violence and Aboriginal leaders active in addressing family violence, sexual assault and child abuse across NSW exemplifies such an approach informed by an understanding of the historical context and its legacies on the current environment in Aboriginal communities.
- In the situation of collective trauma experienced by Australia's Aboriginal people, acknowledgement of the history and ongoing traumatic effects of assimilation policies and practices is crucial if effective action is to be taken to address the legacies of violence and abuse, so evident today.

Part II

Politics and policies within violence, abuse and oppression

6 Feminism(s) and domestic violence within national policy contexts

Ruth Phillips

Democratic governments tend not to respond to the issues of violence, abuse and oppression in a singular way; however, some aspects of violence, abuse and oppression can be clearly delineated as national social policy responses and often the strength and impact of such responses are directly related to the political, social and economic context in which they operate. National social policies, which are manifested in legislative, educational and service responses to certain social problems, reflect not only the political will of a government to address a social problem but also the historical and political will of communities affected by the problem. This type of social policy response is also increasingly occurring at the global level through institutions such as the United Nations (UN) and similarly reflects the concerns of national governments and global social movement communities.

This chapter will explore the role and character of a range of national responses to domestic violence and make links to the wider political and social transformations that have been central to various national contexts. Such transformations include: the historical and current impact of the women's movement and its contribution to social policy within states; progress in democracy; economic development; and, in a number of advanced western democracies, the backlash against feminism that has seen a shift away from a focus on domestic violence as a feminist issue at the national level. A further social transformation that is important at the periphery of the discussion in this chapter but important for many national contexts, is in the global social policy context. At this level there have been two key developments; one, an increasing recognition of domestic violence as a human rights issue and two, international feminist debates related to the critical, contemporary political rift between the West and the Islamic world which raises key tensions for the future of feminist activism and interventions regarding violence against women across diverse cultures.

As a means of exploring the broad scope of change in social policy responses to domestic violence, this chapter first briefly reviews the theoretical importance of feminism in developing national domestic violence policy responses. Second, it examines some national social policy responses to domestic violence in a diverse range of countries.

A discussion about social policy responses to domestic violence in national policy contexts necessitates an engagement with feminism. There is a powerful consistency in how domestic violence was raised as a public policy issue across the world and it would be difficult to deny that the women's movement, the feminist vehicle for social change, has been the key instigator. As will be discussed below, this social policy agenda setting has occurred at different times within different countries and internationally continues to be a dynamic force in women's struggles for security from violence. However, to move forward with the wider discussion of national social policy responses to domestic violence, the contribution of the various feminism have to be noted.

The wide range of feminist theories and practices has resulted in the evolution of various strands of feminism, such as 'liberal feminism, radical feminism, socialist feminism, black feminism, ecofeminism, cultural feminism, political feminism, lesbian feminism, psychoanalytic feminism and academic feminism' (Fawcett, 2000: 2). These distinctions have emerged from both analytic and activist frameworks. A further and highly influential contemporary feminist perspective is postmodern feminism, sometimes seen as the dominant thread of 'third wave feminism' (Howie and Tauchert, 2004; Chesler, 2005). Postmodern feminism has been subject to various interpretations and developments. Emphasis on relativity, pluralism and a dismissal of universally applicable structural criteria has resulted in strong critiques. For some, postmodern feminism is seen to have promoted fragmentation and a rejection of both entrenched structural disadvantage and collective action (Brewer, 2002; Stacey, 1986). However, others have, in various ways, developed forms of what can be called 'critical' postmodernism. Although perspectives vary, these move beyond both modern foundationalism and the plurality and relativity characteristic of postmodernism, to ground discussion about the operation of power imbalances within specific contexts. This in turn facilitates the making of intercontextual comparisons (Fraser and Nicholson, 1993; Fawcett, 2000).

However, debates taking place within the various feminisms do not mean that structural analyses and in particular the notion of patriarchy have disappeared from feminist action and discourses. In the domestic violence service sector across the world there is still a strong presence of radical feminist frameworks as the structural oppression of women is clearly linked to gendered power relations. The increasingly recognized global women's movement appears to reflect an adherence to recognizing the shared effects of men's structural domination across many different cultures and cultural contexts (Antrobus, 2004). However, contemporary feminist language is careful to be inclusive of diversity and difference and has a very strong adherence to broad social justice principles. Key components of this approach are summarized by Antrobus (2004); where she argues for a 'Women, Culture and Development' approach in addressing new challenges and current dilemmas for women. In this she emphasizes the importance of ongoing engagement with issues of class, race/ethnicity and nationality. She also brings to the fore links between production and reproduction and considers matters of power, conflict and the larger social, cultural and political context of women's lives. Antrobus (2004) further stresses the centrality of family, community and religion and draws attention to the importance of women's agency in challenging inequalities.

For this chapter the types of feminisms that are most appropriate in translating policy into action for women affected by violence are located in the diversity of feminist theory outlined above. Although many tensions remain within feminist approaches, it is evident that in each national context in which the state has developed a social policy response to domestic violence, the women's movement, both local and global, has played a key role in placing it on the agenda as an important public policy issue. As Featherstone (2004) noted, there is a necessity for the maintenance of a range of feminist perspectives on domestic violence, both in relation to its historical role in raising it as gendered violence and a form of resistance by women, and as an ongoing discourse. Although the ways in which feminisms have been applied and have contributed to domestic violence policy development within the various states are diverse, the value of the multiplicity of the range of feminisms is central to the notion of 'feminism' in this chapter. In other words, feminisms are most usefully maintained in a national domestic violence policy when their application acknowledges the structural questions, whilst avoiding ideas of women's 'universal' experience of domestic violence. By including postmodern, particularly 'critical postmodern' approaches to this issue, there will be greater understanding of the diverse experiences of women, the ways in which cultural and contextual factors operate and the differing ways of resisting and countering violence.

National domestic violence policies

Domestic violence policies of advanced industrial democracies generally comprise core components for women's security from domestic violence and provide support for women who are experiencing or have experienced domestic violence. This can include: funding and political support for research on the incidence of violence across all communities; conducting broad public education campaigns against violence against women; introducing appropriate civil and criminal legislation against perpetrators of violence and for the protection of women experiencing domestic violence; funding programmes for individual and family support and emergency services and accommodation and; supporting domestic violence education of institutional professionals such as police, medical staff and judges.

In a significant international comparative study of national domestic violence policies in thirty-six countries, Weldon (2002) produced important data about the development of governmental responses to the activism of the women's movement over a twenty-year period. This research provides scope to track state policy responses to the demands of women's movement action on domestic violence. For example in Australia, with a starting point of zero for the number of domestic violence policy areas addressed in 1974, it became a world leader twenty years later, sharing, along with Canada, a position at the top of a domestic violence policy achievements list with seven key areas addressed (Weldon, 2002). This level of policy response fared extremely well in comparison to European welfare states such as Sweden with four and Denmark and Finland with two or the surprising record of Italy, in 1994, which had no governmental policy on violence against women (Weldon, 2002: 30, Table 2.1).

Weldon's (2002) research raises the issue of diverse culture and development in international studies and concludes that although culture and values should not be dismissed in terms of having some impact on government policies relating to violence against women, what is most important is which 'actors and arenas' in each culture matter in relation to women and violence (Weldon, 2002: 37, 195). 'Strong, independently organised women's movements' are not only a key but are a necessary factor in determining improved government responsiveness to violence against women (Weldon, 2002: 195). In most national contexts it is evident that without the women's movement, violence against women would never have been forced out of the private domain on to the public agenda. Weldon's (2002) research reaffirms the importance of the women's movement, but must be seen in the context of the time of the research that relies on data collected up until the mid-1990s. The study did not reflect more recent policy developments in newly democratized states such as South Korea or Taiwan where the women's movement had its first successes in pushing domestic violence policy onto state agendas in the 1990s and later. Further, Weldon's (2002) study was completed in the heyday of women's policy responses by governments that have since experienced both a shift towards more conservative politics and a backlash against feminism, including Australia, the United States, and many European states (Phillips, 2006a; Hannam, 2007).

Shared movements, different contexts and disparate futures

It is not possible to provide a comprehensive overview of all national contexts. The following is a sampling of domestic violence policy responses in different national contexts where domestic violence has been pursued as a key social policy issue to varying degrees at the national level. Most countries have different levels of government and often states or provincial governments within a country may vary in how they respond to domestic violence. Examining national level responses to domestic violence provides an indicator of policy leadership on the issue and a fair overview of what types of resources are allocated to it as a social problem.

It is evident that in most cases where there is strong democratic government, an advanced economy and an active women's movement, the policy responses tend to be stronger. However, regardless of how powerful the policy response has been, there is constant recognition of two key factors. The first is that the level of domestic violence is high everywhere and the second is that states do not provide enough resources to tackle this serious social problem. Many women are still lacking support and protection from violence across the world. This is highlighted in international statistics provided by Amnesty International. Here it is shown that: at least one in every three women or up to one billion women have been beaten, coerced into sex, or otherwise abused in their lifetimes, that up to 70 per cent of female murder victims are killed by their male partners (in Zambia the rate is five women per week and two per week in the UK), that in the Russian Federation 36,000 women are beaten on a daily basis by their husbands, and that in Pakistan 42 per cent of women accept violence as part of their fate (Amnesty International, 2004).

The United Kingdom, Canada and Australia share democratic and parliamentary models, have had Labour Party style governments for significant periods in the last twenty years and are therefore often compared in their responses to social policy issues. As former British colonies, Canada and Australia are settler nations with similarly marginalized Indigenous populations and can often be seen to converge in their social and economic responses to core social policy issues. A shared social transformation in all three countries in relation to domestic violence was the role of the women's movement, in terms of both timing and impact. Indeed, if one compares current commentaries of women's organizations in the three countries, there are ongoing similarities in contemporary concerns about formal state responses to domestic violence as part of the general shift to more conservative and less feminist influenced policy responses. This is clearly expressed in the extract below from a UK women's organization website:

> In the last 8 years the UK Government has introduced new laws and policy initiatives and funding for certain forms of support. This has been matched by research and guidance at a senior level in the police and Crown Prosecution Service. The UK Government has also been active in consulting the voluntary sector on various forms of violence against women.
>
> However the statistics and our experience of working with the women and girls whose lives are damaged by violence demonstrate that this is simply not enough and that UK Government initiatives, whilst welcome, are still failing to adequately protect or support women. In particular UK Government responses have been marked by lack of leadership and joined up working: there is no single lead on all forms of violence against women.
>
> (Campaign, 2006)

It could not be said that there has been progress in the past eight years in Australia. On the contrary, the current, conservative national government has wound back its commitment to women's policy very significantly, and similar failings of policy are evident (Chappell, 2001; Phillips, 2006a; Sawer, 2003; Maddison and Partridge, 2007). These are particularly reflected in a clear 'post-feminist' shift to support for the family as a site to address domestic violence rather than addressing the gendered nature of the violence at a societal level by supporting women's policy input (Phillips, 2006a). Similar to the failures cited above in the UK context, the Australian and Canadian governments also fall short on their funding of policies for women experiencing or escaping violence. In both countries this is most extreme for Indigenous women. Economic and social marginalization and racism are added factors to Indigenous women's vulnerability as is evidenced in the higher rates of violence and in particular, homicides of women in those groups (Australian Productivity Commission, 2003; Canadian

Broadcasting Commission, 2004). There is also evidence that there has been little success in ameliorating the level of violence against women and that public debate and discourses that recognize domestic violence as a problem of gender and power have disappeared off the policy agendas of all three national governments (Phillips, 2006a; Hannam, 2007; Walby and Allen, 2004).

In the United States, where the liberal feminist dominated women's movement saw its most rapid progress in its gender equality claims, there has been a far more varied set of policy responses to violence against women. Federal government initiatives addressing violence against women expanded in the 1990s (in particular the passage of the Violence Against Women Act of 1994) and there is an Office of Violence Against Women in the Federal Department of Justice and an influential National Advisory Committee on Violence Against Women established in 1995, which has a broad policy scope. Although it was a long struggle by women's organizations to achieve serious police intervention across the United States, nearly all states in the USA 'have mandatory arrest policies for felony domestic assaults and warrantless arrest for unwitnessed domestic violence-related misdemeanour assaults'(Bachman, 2003: 11). However, mandatory arrest has not been a consistently successful policy and various researchers have reported police backlashes against the requirement and a high incidence of arrest of victims in the process, leading some feminists to call on governments to spend more money on support services for victims of violence rather than pursuing policy intervention policies (Bachman, 2003).

Having emerged as a democratic state in 1947, Japan was open to influences and social movements from the West at the height of the women's movement of the 1970s. Japanese feminists were active in the early women's liberation movement, instigating campaigns around inequalities in family law, exposing problems for working women and campaigning against sexist advertising (Hannam, 2007). Japanese women established a strong identity with other Asian women and were very active in the international context, drawing attention to the oppression of women in the Philippines, Korea and Indonesia, as well as influencing their own government (Hannam, 2007). Similar women's activism to that in the USA and Europe that called for support for women affected by sexual and domestic violence was also a focus of the movement. However their achievements were minor and by the 1980s little had been achieved by way of support or policy response from governments in Japan (Yoshihama, 2002). Research showed that the issue of domestic violence has been extremely difficult to address in Japan. Data from 1992 showed that 61 per cent of the Japanese population believed that women provoked abuse and around 50 per cent felt that men's use of violence against their female partners could be justified under certain circumstances (Yoshihama, 2002). It is not surprising that in this social context it was not until 2001 that domestic violence prevention laws were passed and that currently governments provide little support for women experiencing violence with this being left up to the private and non-government sectors (Yoshihama, 2002). Most of the support policies adopted by the states mentioned above have, in recent years, been taken up by the private and non-government sectors in Japan; however, more recently some governments have begun to develop policy and to put in place some support services (Yoshihama, 2002). Nonetheless, the current state of support is inadequate, with limited access to shelters and an ongoing resistance to recognizing domestic violence. The courts still accept violence, such as rape in marriage and the welfare system is not able to accommodate victims of domestic violence. According to Yoshihama for things to change in Japan:

> The connection between domestic violence, structural inequality, underlying male supremacy, and women's subordination must be unequivocally recognized. The recognition of these connections must guide the development of policy and services in order to respond to the immediate needs of women, while simultaneously seeking to reform the current framework in an attempt to eradicate domestic violence.
>
> (Yoshihama, 2002: 551)

This reflects a strong feminist analysis of domestic violence policy failure in Japan and, consistent with other states discussed above, the ongoing need to struggle for state recognition of domestic violence as a problem of gender and power, regardless of how advanced the democratic and economic system may be.

In examining state responses to domestic violence in countries with very strong religious dimensions to the operation of the state and society, where economies have been seen as developing for many years and with less developed democratic access to policy change, more extreme but similar problems exist. For example, in India, Pakistan and Sri Lanka, although internationally shared experiences of the types of violence committed against women are evident, it is clear that responses by the state and community discourses highlight distinct historical and local contexts (Goonesekere, 2004). For example, in adherence to traditional religious and cultural practices, acts such as 'dowry deaths' in India and 'stove deaths' (doused in petrol and set alight by family members) (Terzieff, 2002) in Pakistan continue. These constitute extreme forms of domestic violence, where issues of gender and power in the home are played out in the public sphere and where they can be seen as a response to women's improved rights to property and citizenship (Goonesekere, 2004). However, there is diversity in these national contexts, as India has a history equal to its colonizers in women's movement demands since their independence struggles, calling early in the twentieth century for women's suffrage and in the second wave of the movement since the 1970s, for policies addressing violence against women (Hannam, 2007). However, it was not until 2006 that India finally passed national legislation to protect women from domestic violence (Bhat, 2006). Although very pleased with the achievement of this new law which acknowledges the wide range of acts which constitute domestic violence, the women's movement in India is now demanding a commitment from the national government to provide appropriate funding for accommodation for women escaping domestic violence. The need for this action, in turn, reflects further limitations of the government's policy response to domestic violence (Bhat, 2006).

Many African states developed policy responses to domestic violence in the 1990s which vary according to the country's economic and political capacity. The emergence of these policies concur with the postcolonial, post-cold war political environment where there were real opportunities for many African citizens, particularly women, to 'participate, in a serious way, in deciding the legal and constitutional rights of people in their own countries and the desired forms of government' (Mikell, 1995: 409). It was also a period of time when the various women's movements and activists began to identify with feminism (Mikell, 1995), consistent with the emergence of what is termed 'third world' feminism (Mohanty, 2003; Narayan, 1997). In South Africa, for example, the government has put in place many policy commitments based on the Domestic Violence Act (116 of 1998) which aimed to provide legal protection to women, appropriate responses from the police and the courts and to compel agencies across government to provide services and support based on the intent of the Act (Vetten, 2005). As Vetten found in her analysis of how budget allocations were made in response to the demands of the Act, the inadequacy of the financial commitment by the government meant a clear failure to 'back up national constitutional commitments with budgetary commitments' and represents 'one aspect of weak accountability to women' (2005: 292). Although clearly a government engaged with massive social and economic transformations since its democratization in the post-apartheid government, the impact of constraints on financial commitment to policy implementation results in the same types of limitation of support for women described in the above discussion about advanced democracies such as Australia and the United Kingdom.

Implications for human services providers

Although there is ample evidence of the recognition of domestic violence as a serious social problem and social policy issue across all national contexts, what this chapter highlights is a consistency in the limitations and failures of national policy responses. The integral link between women's movements and feminism are also evident across diverse national contexts, acting and struggling within the limitations of the social, economic and political dimensions of a particular national community.

In every national context where women are engaging in mobilization to get their governments to act to protect women from domestic violence and to support women who are experiencing or escaping violence, women are calling for more support and a greater commitment from those governments. This is particularly the case for service providers to women affected by domestic violence. The refrain is repeated over and over, in every national context, that there is an unacceptable level of violence against women and there are not enough resources allocated by government to adequately address the problem. It appears that there is no single example of convergence of all the ingredients required to ensure a comprehensive and effective social policy response to domestic violence, including sufficient services for intervention and victim support.

Based on the commentaries of feminist scholars, researchers and women activists, the ideal national context would require a high level of participation of women in government leadership, a strong, supported women's movement, a large financial commitment by government towards domestic violence programmes, a society prepared to recognize domestic violence as an issue of gender/power relations and the acknowledgement of the importance of equal citizenship and human rights between women and men.

The increasing global response to domestic violence has created a valuable resource of strength for human service providers in this field. As more research is done, culturally specific services are developed and the increased emphasis in human rights is made, the greater the resources are for improving social policy interventions and service models across all countries. The growing voice of the women's movement in developing countries and the more public debates about religious and culturally based oppressions of women in various parts of the world are providing a new context to reassert a feminist analysis and dampen the effects of the backlash against feminism. An interconnected, globalized world also allows for strong social movement responses to borderless exploitations of women such as sex trafficking and, in turn, makes links between the range of types of violence women currently endure.

The short discussion in this chapter about the historical and contemporary differences within feminisms offers a tried and tested paradigm for understanding the prevalence and place of domestic violence across all national contexts. By highlighting feminism's diversity and propensity to transform according to different national contexts and experiences of women, this chapter has highlighted the intrinsic value of feminism as a theoretical and practice framework for producing appropriate social policy response to domestic violence.

Chapter summary

Feminism(s) and domestic violence within national policy contexts

- There is a powerful consistency in how domestic violence was raised as a public policy issue across the world through the women's movement; the feminist vehicle for social change has been the key instigator.
- It is widely agreed that the tensions arising from the developments of postmodern feminism articulated theoretically what many women living outside the dominant middle class, white, heterosexual, able-bodied western women's movement, saw as the failure of the women's movement to be inclusive.
- Domestic violence policies of advanced industrial democracies generally comprise core components for women's security from domestic violence

(Continued)

(Continued)

and provide support for women who are experiencing or have experienced domestic violence.

- In adherence to traditional religious and cultural practices, acts such as 'dowry deaths' in India and 'stove deaths' (doused in petrol and set alight by family members) in Pakistan, which are extreme forms of domestic violence, where issues of gender and power in the home are played out in the public sphere and often linked to men's sense of threat to women's improved rights to property and citizenship, are common.
- Japanese women established a strong identity with other Asian women and were very active in the international context, drawing attention to the oppression of women in the Philippines, Korea and Indonesia, as well as influencing their own government.
- Many African states developed policy responses to domestic violence in the 1990s; these vary according to the country's economic and political capacity.
- Although there is ample evidence of the recognition of domestic violence as a serious social problem and social policy issue across all national contexts, what this chapter highlights is a consistency in the limitations and failures of national policy responses.
- The ideal national context would require a high level of participation of women in government leadership, a strong, supported women's movement, a large financial commitment by government towards domestic violence programmes, a society prepared to recognize domestic violence as an issue of gender/power relations and the acknowledgement of the importance of *equal* citizenship and human rights between women and men.

7 'Violence', criminal justice, the law, policy and practice

Lesley Laing

As discussed in previous chapters, largely in response to calls by feminists, western governments have become increasingly involved over the last thirty years in responding to forms of violence and abuse that are commonly referred to as sexual and domestic violence against women. These forms of violence and abuse are characterized by the fact that they are commonly perpetrated against women, not by strangers, but by known men (Hanmer and Itzin, 2000). In the ensuing years, a wide range of policy and practice responses have been implemented, incorporating reforms and initiatives across diverse domains such as community based women's services and the legal, health, housing and child protection sectors. These include, for example, the establishment of crisis accommodation and support for women escaping domestic violence, the development of specialist counselling and advocacy services for victims/survivors of sexual and domestic violence, the promotion of coordinated interagency or 'joined-up' responses (James-Hanman, 2000) and the implementation of policies that aim to increase recognition by health services of the effects of victimization that are commonly manifested in a range of physical and mental health presentations (Itzin, 2006). This chapter focuses on legal responses to violence against women because these have been at the core of policy responses. Historically,[1] the division between the spheres of 'private' and 'public' life meant that the state was reluctant to intervene in violence against women (Fineman and Mykitiuk, 1994). Hence a key demand of feminist activists was that violence committed within the privacy of intimate relationships be treated in the same way as violence committed in public, that is, as criminal behaviour (Epstein, 1999). Following on from the chapter by Phillips and taking the example of domestic violence, using feminist analysis as a point of critique, this chapter explores the extent to which legal remedies have achieved the core goals of domestic violence policy: increasing the safety of women and holding the perpetrators of violence and abuse accountable (Goodman and Epstein, 2005; Pence and McDonnell, 1999). It will be seen that

---

1 It has recently been argued by Bevacqua and Baker (2004) that the private/public ideology continues to shield men from being held accountable by the law for violence against women.

using the law to address domestic violence has proved more complex and challenging than originally anticipated (Belknap and Potter, 2005; Das Gupta, 2003). The chapter will also attempt to make sense of the challenges that have arisen in attempts to use the law and to identify ways forward.

As highlighted in a number of chapters in this book, definitions of domestic violence are contested. However, the core dynamic of domestic violence is the imposition of a regime of coercive control (Dutton and Goodman, 2005; Herman, 1992; Mahoney, 1991) through a complex pattern of tactics including, but far from limited to, physical and sexual violence, psychological, verbal and financial abuse, social isolation, threats and harming children. This element of coercive control differentiates domestic violence as discussed in this chapter from mutual physical aggression between partners, sometimes referred to as 'common couple violence' (Johnson, 1995), a form of violence measured by crime surveys that has fuelled an ongoing debate about whether domestic violence is gendered (Bagshaw and Chung, 2000; R.P. Dobash, Dobash, Wilson and Daly, 1992).

As has been discussed elsewhere, second wave feminism defined domestic violence as an expression of unequal gender power relations, embedded in historical, social and political contexts that support greater male power and access to resources (Bird, 2004; Stark, 2004). The element of intentionality was also emphasized: 'Violence is seen as intentional behaviour chosen by men as a tactic or resource associated with attempts to control and dominate women' (R.E. Dobash and Dobash, 1992: 248). Subsequent developments within feminism such as challenges by black women to the centralizing of gender as the key lens for exploring women's experiences (hooks, 1981, 1984; Lucashenko, 1994) have extended this understanding of domestic violence by highlighting the ways in which other dimensions of women's lives such as class, race, immigration status, ability and sexuality, 'intersect' (Crenshaw, 1991) with gender to shape women's experiences of violence and of intervention (Almeida and Durkin, 1999; Bograd, 1999). The focus of this chapter is violence against women by current or former intimate male partners, the most prevalent form of domestic violence. However, it is recognized that intimate partner abuse can occur in lesbian relationships. Postmodern feminist critiques have identified the limitations of categories that marginalize and silence women who experience violence and abuse within lesbian relationships (e.g. Ristock, 2002). Readers are referred to the chapter by Irwin for detailed discussion of this topic.

Legal responses to domestic violence

Efforts to address domestic violence through legal reform have targeted both civil and criminal law (NSW Domestic Violence Committee, 1989). The criminal law is concerned with violence that has already been enacted and responds with goals that can be summarized as punishment, deterrence and rehabilitation of the offender (Lewis, Dobash, Dobash and Cavanagh, 2000). In contrast, civil law remedies aim to prevent future violence by placing limitations on the behaviours of the man through the issuing of protection orders, which have various names in different jurisdictions (e.g. restraining orders). These two legal approaches potentially offer complementary assistance to women dealing with violence because together they address both women's safety and perpetrator accountability. However, in most jurisdictions, either one of these approaches to using the law has tended to dominate. In the United States, for example, criminal law policies have been extensively taken up, spurred by the passing of the Violence Against Women Act in 1994 (Das Gupta, 2003; Hanna, 1998).

Using civil law to address domestic violence

In contrast, Australian states and territories (apart from the Australian Capital Territory) have tended until very recently[2] to emphasize civil protection orders as the primary legal response to domestic violence, albeit while endorsing the policy position that 'domestic violence is a crime' (Holder, 2004). It is argued that civil protection orders provide an option for women who may not want their partners prosecuted, nor necessarily to separate from them, but who want the violence to stop (Queensland Domestic Violence Task Force, 1988). Others argue that civil remedies are an inadequate response by the state to the call by feminist activists to treat 'private' violence as a crime, and that this policy approach effectively amounts to the decriminalization of violence committed by intimate partners (McGregor and Hopkins, 1991; Scutt, 2006). Some evidence in support of this argument is found in a recent study in the Australian State of Queensland where Douglas and Godden (2003) reviewed 694 files involving applications for Domestic Violence Protection Orders in the Brisbane Magistrates Court. Despite the files containing evidence of serious violence, such as the use of weapons (22.7 per cent), death threats (15.6 per cent) and visible injuries (37 per cent), only three matters were the subject of a criminal prosecution.

Potential strengths of civil protection orders in making legal protection accessible to women lie in the fact that they can be obtained quickly via interim orders in comparison to slower moving criminal justice processes; that the standard of proof required is the 'balance of possibilities' rather than the higher criminal standard of 'beyond reasonable doubt'; that the conditions placed upon the man can be tailored to the woman's particular situation; and that, in all Australian jurisdictions, breaching the conditions of a protection order constitutes a criminal offence (Putt and Higgins, 1997). The following examples from Australian research, however, illustrate some of the challenges faced by women seeking protection through the civil law.

Although the effectiveness of protection orders rests on the willingness of police to enforce them (Epstein, 1999), a frequent problem identified by victims

---

2 However there has been a recent trend to increased emphasis on the use of the criminal law in states that have undertaken major domestic violence policy review within the last 5 years, for example Tasmania and Victoria.

of domestic violence and their advocates is the failure of police to respond when civil orders are violated (Peirce, 2005). A study by the New South Wales Bureau of Crime Statistics and Research found that police took no action in response to 73.2 per cent of the breaches reported to them (Trimboli and Bonney, 1997). Katzen (2000) studied police responses to violations of protection orders in rural New South Wales and found that police were reluctant to respond to breaches of orders when these occurred in the context of child contact and family law proceedings – even when violence was witnessed by police in contact handovers at the police station – because these were seen as 'family' (private) rather than 'police' (criminal) matters. Also in New South Wales, Edwards (2004) studied protection orders granted in two local courts that included the condition that the man leave the home, termed 'exclusion orders''. She found that, in contested matters, magistrates focused decision-making on the property rights and accom- modation needs of the man; in contrast, none addressed the needs of children. Ironically, the availability of crisis refuges for women and children, the victims of violence, rendered their homelessness invisible to the court. These findings highlight the endurance in the legal system of notions of the family as a private domain and the reluctance to challenge male power therein.

Using the criminal law to address domestic violence

Considerable research and reform effort has focused on the police response to domestic violence because of their crucial role as gatekeepers to the criminal jus- tice system (Robinson and Stroshine, 2005). Prior to the changes instituted through the activism of feminists in the 1960s and 1970s, reluctance by police to treat domestic violence as criminal behaviour reflected the state's historical stance that condoned male violence and control within intimate relationships. Lutze and Symons identify this as the first of three stages in the development of domestic violence policy, which they characterize as 'male privilege and the right to discipline' (Lutze and Symons, 2003: 320). The adoption of policies of pre- ferred or mandatory arrest has been the most common policy response to police resistance to treating domestic assault in the same way as violence committed in other contexts (Hanna, 1998). These policies make arrest the required or pre- ferred police response to domestic assault where there is 'probable cause' to believe that a crime has been committed, whatever the wishes of the victim in the situation (Coker, 2001). The rationale behind such policies is that they remove the discretion of police, thus overcoming attitudes that blame women for their victimization or that minimize violence committed within intimate relationships (Ferraro and Pope, 1993).

Subsequent reform efforts turned to other stages of the criminal justice process such as prosecution in order to redress the historical failure to prosecute domestic assaults. While there is considerable variation in the extent to which domestic violence matters are aggressively prosecuted, under the most extreme, 'hard no drop' prosecution policies: 'Decisions to prosecute are based on the quality of the evidence and the seriousness of the case ... this policy ultimately gives the women no right to choose whether the state criminally prosecutes her partner' (Hanna, 1996: 1867–8). In some jurisdictions, this means that women can be sub-poenaed to appear as witnesses and can be imprisoned if they fail to comply. Hanna (1996) argues that this policy takes the burden of prosecution from the victim, thus removing the incentive for the perpetrator to try to intimidate her and that it meets the demand by feminists that the state not condone domestic violence. Lutze and Symons (2003) characterize this second period of policy development as one of 'male power and the right to protect', in which: 'The very system that inherently protected the privilege of men to discipline their wives would now be mobilized to protect the lives and rights of women ... Domestic violence would be mandated into extinction' (Lutze and Symons, 2003: 322–3).

However, as the following discussion will highlight, criminal justice reforms have not necessarily achieved the aim of having domestic violence treated in the same way as other criminal offences. Further, the following examples will demonstrate that the very reform efforts initiated to assist women have had unintended, negative effects in the lives of some women. Changing police culture has proved a complex and challenging task (Brunetto and Farr-Wharton, 2005; Ferraro and Pope, 1993) and some studies have shown that rates of arrest have not necessarily increased to any great extent in preferred and mandatory arrest jurisdictions (Belknap and Potter, 2005; Lutze and Symons, 2003; Stark, 2004). With respect to prosecution, two studies in the United Kingdom, although conducted almost ten years apart, found that domestic violence cases continue to be treated differently by prosecutors (Cammiss, 2006; Cretney and Davis, 1997). Both studies found that, when cases of domestic and non-domestic assault were compared, despite similarities in the seriousness of the assaultive behaviour, domestic violence cases were more commonly heard in the lower than the higher courts. This reduces the level of penalty that can be applied and also requires the prosecutor to present a version of the assault that can diminish its seriousness (Cammiss, 2006). As a consequence, the woman's account is not fully heard by the court and the true extent and nature of violence against women remains hidden.

At the same time, there is evidence from the United States that policies that require women's 'mandated participation' (Hanna, 1996: 1857) in the criminal justice process, intended to reduce this differential response, have in some cases resulted in unintended, negative consequences. One of the most concerning of these is the increase in numbers of women arrested in jurisdictions with mandatory arrest policies (Raphael, 2004), despite research indicating that most women who use violence are acting in self-defence or in response to an ongoing situation of domestic violation (Miller, 2001). Arrest can make women ineligible to receive victim services, can disadvantage them in child custody and child protection proceedings and can result in loss of employment, rendering them more dependent on their abusers (Coker, 2004; McDermott and Garofalo, 2004). Of particular concern is the potentially disproportionate impact of such policies on the women who are most vulnerable to domestic violence and least resourced to deal with it, such as women marginalized by poverty, race, ethnicity and immigration status (Coker, 2001; Mills, 2003). However, Stark (2004) argues with respect to race, that the evidence to support such concern is not yet available, and that discrimination against people on the basis of race continues to take the form of failing to offer legal protection to certain groups, rather than over-intrusion by criminal justice agencies.

Another negative consequence of efforts to criminalize domestic violence through 'mandatory' policies is the punitive and victim blaming responses to which women that are reluctant to pursue a matter fully through the criminal justice process may be subjected. Such women are often viewed by actors in the justice system through a lens that shapes the problem as one of the 'uncooperative' or 'ambivalent' domestic violence victim/witness. It is frequently assumed that this reluctance to proceed is due to the woman's psychological problems arising from the experience of domestic violence, such as 'learned helplessness' and 'battered women's syndrome' (Walker, 1977–8, 1984). This perspective discourages actors in the justice system from exploring what it is about the system itself that may present impediments to women seeking assistance from it.

When the light is turned onto the system itself, a different picture emerges. For example, a number of studies indicate that victim reluctance is not necessarily the reason that a case fails to proceed: poor police briefs of evidence (Ferraro and Pope, 1993) and failure to notify women of court dates in a timely manner (Keys Young, 2000) are also factors. Research into women's experiences of attempting to use the justice system has found that situational factors such as level of abuse experienced and level of tangible social support (such as help with transport, emergency money and child care), together with systemic barriers such as the lack of accurate and timely information, frustration at the slowness of the system, the cancellation of proceedings and the experience of pressure rather than support by legal personnel, are more predictive of women's decisions to proceed with the legal process than are psychological factors, such as depression (Bennett, Goodman and Dutton, 1999; Fleury-Steiner, Bybee, Sullivan, Belknap and Melton, 2006; Goodman, Bennett and Dutton, 1999).

Most importantly, blaming women for failure to cooperate obscures the evidence that, even if a woman 'cooperates' and follows through with a criminal prosecution, the legal system cannot guarantee to protect her from further violence by the perpetrator either during or after the process (Fleury-Steiner *et al.*, 2006; Ford and Regoli, 1993). From this perspective, the complexity of women's decision-making and the 'calculated risk' (Coker, 2001: 826) she takes in using, not using or using the criminal law only to a certain point, can be better understood.

Evidence of unintended consequences such as these has fuelled debate about the emphasis that should be placed on legal responses to domestic violence. For example, Linda Mills (1999) argues that mandatory policies are incompatible with the feminist goal of empowering women because they override women's decisions and in so doing, replicate the disrespectful, emotionally abusive and coercive behaviour of the domestic violence perpetrator. However, most are reluctant to abandon efforts to use the law and to return to a situation where police and courts ignore domestic violence and treat it as a personal, psychological issue, rather than as an issue of the abuse of power located within a social and historical context that condones male violence against female partners (Epstein, Bell and Goodman, 2003; Stark, 2004).

An impossible task?

What was initially seen as a victory by activists who mobilized to address domestic violence – making 'public' violence committed within the 'privacy' of the family by harnessing the power of the law – has resulted in unintended and harmful consequences for some women. The law continues to fail to hold many men accountable for violence committed in the private sphere, or efforts to force institutional change at a minimum risk pathologizing women and at worst risk harming women who do not accept the 'protection' of the legal system.

To some extent, these difficulties can be seen as a product of the lack of fit between the complexities of domestic violence and the operation of the traditional criminal justice system. For example, the criminal justice system is incident-specific, with only some behaviour defined as falling within its boundaries (Ursel, 2002). Hence only some elements of women's experience are dealt with by the legal system, removed from the core context of the perpetrator's tactics of coercive control. Stark calls this: 'a gross trivialization of the tactics deployed in most cases of battering.' (Stark, 2004: 1317). Prosecution of the perpetrator by the state also conflates the power of the victim with that of the state, rendering invisible the ongoing risk to the safety of the woman when she invokes the criminal law to deal with violence (Romkens, 2006). In addition, the primary focus of the criminal justice system on the perpetrator creates an imbalance in the goals of domestic violence intervention, with offender accountability being emphasized to a greater extent than victim safety (Goodman and Epstein, 2005).

Women call the police for a complex range of reasons (Hoyle and Sanders, 2000) but do not usually envisage becoming involved in a long and complex prosecution process in which they have little control over the outcome, yet where they have much at stake (Bennett *et al.*, 1999). Research into the ways in which women deal with domestic violence reveals that they resist the perpetrator's violence and control in their intimate relationships, albeit in ways that may not be visible to outside observers (Campbell, Rose, Kub and Nedd, 1998; Chantler, 2006; Davies *et al.*, 1998; Lempert, 1996). However, women's strategies of resistance are constrained by factors that include the coercive control that the perpetrator strives to impose, her access to resources, the often disappointing response she receives from formal and informal supports and her social location (Anderson and Saunders, 2003; Baker, 1997; Cavanagh, 2003; Dutton, 1996; Schneider, 1992). From this perspective, a woman's use of the law can be seen as merely one of many ongoing strategies she may choose over time in efforts to increase her safety and that of her children (Lewis *et al.*, 2000). Against this context, arrest and criminal prosecution will represent narrow options for many women who are grappling with complex choices. Unfortunately, negative inter-actions with criminal justice personnel may deter women from pursuing legal remedies at a future time (Fleury-Steiner *et al.*, 2006).

For many feminists, dilemmas and challenges such as those discussed in this chapter are inevitable when a social movement such as the one against domestic violence engages with the patriarchal state in order to bring about institutional reform (e.g. Ferraro and Pope, 1993; Lutze and Symons, 2003). From this per-spective, engagement with the state to hold men accountable for their violence inevitably reproduces male dominance and their right to discipline women (Lutze and Symons, 2003). Having condoned for centuries men's right to control and discipline wives who do not conform to the dominant view of a dutiful wife, the state's actors in turn discipline those women who do not conform to the domi-nant view of the 'worthy, cooperative victim'. Thus women who fight back against their abusers may be arrested and women who choose not to proceed with the state's prosecution of their partner or ex-partner can be imprisoned or their claims for protection at a future time may be callously rejected because they are judged 'uncooperative'. Coker (2001) argues that feminist domestic violence policy has overestimated the power of the state to assist abused women, while simultaneously underestimating the power of state to harm them. Hence she cau-tions that: 'in developing anti-domestic violence strategies, we must attend to the coercive power of the state, as well as the coercive power of battering men' (Coker, 2001: 860).

Coker's argument is consistent with the problematizing of the second wave fem-inist public/private dichotomy by feminists who locate themselves within a post-colonial worldview and who critique second wave feminism for failing to address white privilege and thus marginalizing the experiences of many women (for example, hooks, 1981; Pewewardy, 2004). Almeida and colleagues (1994) argue:

> While privatization is the fundamental tool of patriarchal oppression within a white, heterosexual relationship ... racial and homosexual oppression begin as public events ... Subjected to public displays of humiliation, mar-ginalization, bigotry and hatred, the intimate relationships of heterosexuals of color and homosexuals of all races are undermined and rendered invisi-ble by public policies and the absence of supports.
>
> (Almeida, Woods, Messineo, Font, and Heer, 1994: 102)

Failure to account for these differences in the experience of oppression can be understood from this perspective to offer an explanation for the limitations of a change agenda based on making 'private' violence a 'public' crime. Such poli-cies can result in harmful intrusions of the state into the lives of women who are already experiencing (often unacknowledged) oppressions in the public realm.

In Australia, Carole Bacchi (1999a) agrees that engagement with the state was necessary if the issue of 'private violence' was to be made 'public', and argues that this necessarily 'shap[es] the forms of "public" recognition that are available' (Bacchi, 1999: 173). Hence, treating domestic assault in the same way as common assault was the most obvious option, yet the consequences, as outlined above, were not what feminist activists anticipated. Bacchi's (1999b) 'what's the problem (represented to be)' approach to analysing social policy is useful in making sense of these unanticipated outcomes. While not discounting the work of feminist activism in bringing to light the worrying conditions of women's lives, Bacchi does not see social problems such as domestic violence as existing 'out there' awaiting discovery. Rather, she understands policies as 'constituting competing interpretations or representations of political issues' (Bacchi, 1999: 2).

These representations include solutions and can be interrogated to discover their material effects, such as those discussed in this chapter. Bacchi's approach to policy analysis draws attention to the assumptions, gaps and limitations in problem representations. In this approach, the role of context is crucial, because this shapes the forms that such problem representations can take.

Bacchi's (1999b) perspective can assist in understanding why shaping the problem of domestic violence as a criminal issue has been more vigorously taken up in the United States than in other western nations. Framing domestic violence as a criminal problem fits well in a context in which policies that are 'tough on crime' have considerable political appeal (Coker, 2001; Snider, 1998). The United States is a country which is characterized by emphasis on the free market economy and a residual approach to welfare provision, marked in recent years by increasing limitations on the availability of welfare support (Peter, 2006). In this context, alternate representations of domestic violence, such as a problem of women's unequal access to material resources, are less likely to be taken up. This is a point made by Coker (2001) who contrasts the ready legislative support for high levels of funding for criminal responses to domestic violence in the United States with the reluctance to allocate funds to measures that would make women both less vulnerable to domestic violence and better able to deal with it, such as education, job training, access to legal aid, emergency and long-term housing.

Coker offers an alternate representation in suggesting that a 'material resources test' be applied to the development of all domestic violence policies (Coker, 2000: 1009). Such a test would prioritize domestic violence law reform and other policies that improve women's access to material resources. She argues that this would put considerations of the 'intersectionality' (Crenshaw, 1991) of gender, class and race at the forefront rather than at the margins of policy development. Coker's suggested approach would address the charge by critics of domestic violence policies that 'strategies of criminalization have benefited privileged white women at the expense of women of colour, aboriginal and immigrant women' (Snider, 1998: 3).

In making this suggestion, Coker is drawing on a wealth of research that indicates that access to material resources both affects women's vulnerability to domestic violence and constrains their attempts to deal with it (e.g. AIHW *et al.*, 2006; Anderson and Saunders, 2003; Sullivan and Bybee, 1999). This stands in contrast to the inconsistent and contested research findings about the effectiveness of arrest in preventing future domestic violence (Garner and Maxwell, 2000; Weisz, 2001). Nevertheless, the uptake of mandatory and preferred arrest policies in the United States has continued.

Reservations by British feminists about the direction of current domestic violence policy under New Labour exemplify both the limitations of representations of domestic violence as primarily a criminal problem and the political struggle that the feminist movement faces in arguing for broader representations (e.g. Ball and Charles, 2006; Harwin, 2006). Under the Domestic Violence, Crime and Victims Act which became law in England and Wales in late 2004, domestic violence is recognized as a priority issue and located within a crime reduction framework. Some important initiatives are included, such as making a breach of non-molestation (protection) orders a criminal offence. However, many reforms advocated by feminist domestic violence groups were not included: no additional funding was allocated to women's refuges and advocacy services; the issue of safe child contact was not addressed; and a gender neutral definition of domestic violence was adopted (Harwin, 2006). Thus, tactical framing of domestic violence to fit broader policy frames brings both gains and losses: 'in the process more radical feminist definitions of the issues are marginalized and the goal of empowering women and challenging gendered power relations and the unequal distribution of resources between men and women is sidelined' (Ball and Charles, 2006: 182).

Carole Smart's (1989) analysis of the ways in which the law exercises power is also useful in understanding the struggle that domestic violence activists have encountered in seeking to use the law to empower the victims of domestic violence. She argues that the law's resistance to feminist challenge and its disqualification of women's experience/knowledge arises from its harnessing of two parallel mechanisms of power:

> If we accept that the law, like science, makes a claim to truth and that this is indivisible from the exercise of power, we can see that the law exercises power not simply in its material effects (judgements) but also in its ability to disqualify other knowledges and experiences. Non-legal knowledge is therefore suspect and/or secondary.
>
> (Smart, 1989: 11)

Smart's work helps us to understand why interagency or 'joined up' approaches, at once so commonly urged in responding to complex issues such as domestic violence, are so difficult to implement. Many initiatives that aim to make the criminal justice process more responsive to women's complex needs are located within interagency partnerships between legal and social service agencies. Lutze and Symons (2003: 324) characterize this as the third phase of domestic violence policy development, one of 'collaborative empowerment'. They identify as the biggest challenge in collaboration between social service and criminal justice agencies, the need to 'equalise the power between the agencies' (Lutze and

Symons, 2003: 324). In this endeavour, the greater power of the criminal justice agencies is seen as the biggest obstacle.

Romkens (2006) provides a case study of the ways in which the criminal justice system positions itself as central within domestic violence interagency initiatives. The collaborative programme in this case aimed to provide women being stalked by ex-partners with protection through electronic alarms. In order to be accepted into the program, women were required to demonstrate both prior and future willingness to engage with the legal system. The criteria for eligibility included the requirements that the woman have a civil protection order, that she be willing to give evidence in the event of an arrest, and that she be assessed as at high risk, based on her ex-partner's criminal record. As has already been discussed, women may have many valid reasons for not pursuing legal solutions to domestic violence. Although the women's narratives, elicited thorough comprehensive assessment interviews with social workers revealed that all applicants for the programme had suffered severe and chronic violence, three-quarters of the women were either rejected or withdrew their applications to join the programme because they could not meet the legal criteria for entry. The women's accounts were seen as 'subjective' and given less priority than the legal criteria that made claims to 'objectivity'. Among those disproportionately excluded were immigrant women, a vulnerable group with least access to other resources for protection. Echoing Lutze and Symonds (2003), Romkems advises against collaborative endeavours that do not take account of the operations of power between the various players:

> The results presented here point toward a paradoxical dynamic that developed at the crossroads of collaboration between the criminal legal system and other disciplines. The legal system operated as a powerful and superior gatekeeper, precisely at a time when a range of professionals are invited to support and improve protection of victims.
>
> (Romkens, 2006: 176)

Implications for human service professionals

Findings from research such as that cited in this chapter about the unintended and unanticipated consequences of attempts to use the legal system to assist women dealing with domestic violence have encouraged a range of initiatives that aim to make the criminal justice system more responsive to the struggles of women dealing with domestic violence. For example Epstein and colleagues (2003) advocate an approach termed 'prosecution in context' in which the prosecutor retains discretion about the decision to prosecute but the complex context of women's lives is taken into account in decisions about proceeding. Key to this approach is the provision of intensive advocacy/support services that are independent of the prosecution so that women receive support that is long-term and not limited to assistance in navigating the legal system. Other initiatives include specialist domestic violence courts (Eley, 2005; Wittner, 1998) and policing approaches that view a positive police response more broadly than as simply arrest (Holder, 2001). For example, a woman's contact with police can be an entry point to a range of information and support services (Hoyle and Sanders, 2000).

Initiatives such as these are underpinned by a number of core principles derived from the research cited in this chapter. Most importantly, new policies that draw more women into contact with the legal system must be accompanied by the provision of specialist women's domestic violence support and advocacy services (Epstein, 1999; Pence and McDonnell, 1999; Ursel, 2002). These services can support women as they attempt to navigate complex and confusing legal processes and can identify situations in which women are being harmed by procedures intended to assist them. In addition, the possibility of unintended consequences from all initiatives requires a commitment to ongoing evaluation of domestic violence policy and practice. This evaluation needs to focus on process as well as outcomes (such as arrest and prosecution rates) in order to ensure that the voices of women attempting to use the law are centralized (Erez and Belknap, 1998; Lewis,, 2004; Lewis *et al.*, 2000).

In conclusion, this chapter has explored some of the challenges involved in attempting to use the law to address domestic violence. A range of theoretical frameworks have been applied to help to unpack the unexpected challenges and unintended consequences that have arisen as part of this endeavour. With some limited exceptions (for example, Mills, 2003), few advocate totally repudiating efforts to use the law to respond to domestic violence. However, as research into domestic violence increases our understanding of its complexity and of women's responses to it, it is clear that legal responses alone are inadequate. In finding new ways forward, the initial focus on the operations of power between perpetrator and victim must be expanded to include critical reflection on the operations of power between women in different social locations, between women seeking help and those responding and between the many agencies that are involved in intervening.

Chapter summary

'Violence', criminal justice, the law, policy and practice

- Legal responses to violence against women, including domestic violence, have been at the core of policy responses initiated by second wave feminist activists in order to challenge the reluctance of the state to intervene in the 'private' realm of the family. However, using both the civil and criminal law to increase the safety of women and to hold perpetrators accountable, has proved more complex and challenging than originally anticipated.
- While civil law remedies potentially offer the advantages of accessibility, speed and flexibility, they may fail to hold perpetrators accountable for what are criminal behaviours and women's safety may be jeopardized by failure of police to act on breaches of protection orders.

(Continued)

- Criminal justice reforms such as polices of 'mandatory' arrest and prose-cution have not necessarily achieved the aim of having domestic assaults treated in the same way as other criminal assaults. Further, the very reforms that aimed to assist women have at times had unintended, negative effects in the lives of women, particularly women who are most vulnera-ble to domestic violence and least resourced to deal with it, such as women marginalized by poverty, race, ethnicity and immigration status.
- The research evidence suggests that future efforts to enhance legal reme-dies for domestic violence need to be grounded in understandings of the complexity of women's responses to domestic violence, such that a woman's use of the law is merely one of many, ongoing strategies she may choose over time in efforts to increase her safety and that of her children. Further, the possibility of unintended consequences from all initiatives requires a commitment to ongoing evaluation that focuses on process from the woman's perspective as well as on legal outcomes.
- A range of feminist theoretical perspectives – radical, postcolonial and postmodern – offer insights into the outcomes of efforts to use the law to address domestic violence. These highlight that the initial focus on the operations of power between perpetrator and victim must be expanded to include critical reflection on the operations of power between women in different social locations, between women seeking help and those respond-ing and between the many agencies that are involved in intervening.

8 Challenging the second closet

Intimate partner violence between lesbians

Jude Irwin

Publicly addressing the issue of lesbian battering, while necessary, is done with the recognition that we live in increasingly repressive times. The hard won gains of the civil rights movement, women's movement and gay and lesbian rights movement over the past twenty five years have been met by increasing resistance and setbacks. Many lesbians are understandably reluctant to air issues related to lesbian battering, for fear of triggering homophobic attacks on our communities. In a society where there has been no acceptance of lesbian relationships, the fears are legitimate. By discussing these issues openly we risk further repression. Yet our only alternative is one of silence, a silence that traps battered lesbians into believing they are alone and that there are no resources available to them.

(Lobel, 1986: 7)

Lesbian relationship violence remains an albatross to the battered women's movement recognised as something we must deal with eventually but not fully embraced in research, theorising or action.

(Ristock, 2002: 8)

Feminist activism, practice and research has played a key role in exposing violence against women and children (Genovese, 2000; Kelly, 1988; MacKinnon, 1982; Millett, 1970; Mitchell, 1971; Walker, 1990; Walby, 1990). The two quotes above, written over fifteen years apart, show that although lesbians began to speak out about the violence in their relationships in the early 1980s it still remains difficult to acknowledge. Why is there such reticence and ambivalence about acknowledging and responding to intimate partner violence between lesbians? How does this ambivalence work to conceal the violence? What impact does this silencing have on lesbians' experiences of intimate partner violence in their relationships? and on the responses of others to this violence?

In this chapter I address these questions by showing how heteronormative assumptions and understandings related to domestic violence (intimate partner violence) have produced and reinforced the invisibility of intimate partner violence between lesbians. The last three decades have seen feminists' engagement in practices of naming and producing discourses on male violence while, at the same time, working to relocate it in the political context. Second wave feminists have refigured the family as a site of patriarchal power relations (see for example Kelly, 1988; Dobash and Dobash, 1992). They named domestic violence and child abuse as practices of male domination, and control of women and children within familial relations where men were seen as individual agents/enforcers as evidence of a broader dominating patriarchal social order (Genovese, 2000). In doing so they have posed challenges to dominant discourses which had previously legitimized and naturalized intimate partner violence. They also critiqued the once unproblematic distinction between the public and private, destabilizing the concept of the home as the uncontested space for male control, reframing it as a public rather than a private concern. These challenges have played a crucial role in influencing how violence against women has been theorized. Different theorising has produced powerful discourses (knowledge and practice), that both describe the effects of violence and are also productive of very real effects (Weedon, 1987). These have become powerful social practices which simultaneously constitute understandings both about domestic violence and the people involved. In this chapter I reflect on how the development of discourses surrounding domestic violence have influenced and produced particular understandings of intimate partner violence between lesbians. I consider critiques, debates and dissenting voices within early radical, lesbian cultural and radical lesbian feminisms and argue that the theorizing about domestic violence has produced particular conceptions, unintentionally shaping the invisibility of intimate partner violence between lesbians. I argue that within both policy and practice contexts, the privileging of heteronormative assumptions related to domestic violence both establishes and produces invisibility of domestic violence between lesbians. I draw on stories of lesbians who have experienced intimate partner violence to show that while they may encounter similar forms of abuse in their relationships to those encountered by heterosexual women, the heteronormative discursive constitutions of intimate partner violence generate and limit understandings and responses to violence in their lives, accentuating its obscurity.

Second wave feminisms' theorizing of male violence against women

Although the contribution of second wave feminisms has been discussed in other chapters in this book, a brief overview at this stage is also necessary here in order to locate intimate partner violence between lesbians within the wider frame. As has become clear, feminisms, similar to other grand or meta theories in the late 1960s and early 1970s, posited various explanations and solutions for the transformation of humanity. Although there were substantial differences within second wave feminisms, the broad focus was on establishing causes and consequences of women's oppression and prescribing strategies for women's liberation. This involved: framing ideas with the conventional parameters of logic, reason and coherence; articulating large-scale plans for social change; challenging the assumptions of men's superiority and women's inferiority; cataloguing the effects of gender oppression; reframing dominant discourses about gender, biology and sex; and attempting to live consistently within a chosen feminist perspective (Fraser, 2002).

Early feminist theorizing around women's oppression did not initially conceptualize violence as being integral to patriarchal power; however, with time it became far more implicated in the production and maintenance of patriarchy. In reviewing feminist theoretical explanations of male violence against women in the 1970s, Anne Edwards (1987) asserted that the role violence was seen to play in women's oppression went through significant shifts and, over time, became more integral in the analysis of patriarchy. She suggested that in the early period of the second wave feminist movement two main sources of literature emerged. These were the classical texts of modern (western) feminism and feminist analyses of male violence (Edwards, 1987). The classical texts focused on women's oppression under patriarchy with male dominance seen as being dependent on social, economic, political and ideological structures and although violence was not positioned as central, it was acknowledged as playing a part in sustaining women's oppression (see for example Firestone, 1970; Millett, 1970; Rowbottom, 1973; Mitchell, 1971; De Beauvoir, 1974). Men's domination of women, institutionalized in the patriarchal family and marriage, was exposed and along with this came the threat or possibility of violence. As the impact of patriarchy in all areas of women's lives was being examined, challenges emerged to the taken-for-granted assumptions that had reinforced women's subservient roles and which were therefore important to the maintenance of society.

The feminist analyses of male violence, originally generated by early radical feminist activists, focused on particular forms of violence such as rape (Brownmiller, 1975; Griffin, 1979). In these analyses violence was constituted as having a much more central role in both the production and sustaining of women's oppression. It was within this context of women's oppression that theorizing about violence was further developed, explaining how various forms of violence worked to reinforce women's subjugation and how men's control of women's sexuality for male pleasure played an integral part in sustaining this oppression. Edwards argued that the later analyses of male violence developed theoretical perspectives encompassing all forms of male violence, abuse and exploitation, linking it to an overall system of male dominance with sexuality having a pivotal role in the maintenance of women's subordination with sexual difference being seen as the origin of women's oppression (see for example Daly, 1973, 1978; Dworkin, 1981; MacKinnon, 1982; Barry, 1979; Rich, 1980). It was only when women were liberated from the sex/class system that all other forms of oppression would be addressed (Daly, 1978; Dworkin, 1981; MacKinnon, 1982).

As radical feminists scrutinized the part sexuality played in sustaining women's subjugation, aggression and the need for men to dominate were seen to be a normal aspect of male sexuality, naturalizing it in other contexts. They drew attention to both the ways in which social and cultural structures and processes defined, shaped and constrained sexuality (both male and female) and how dominant ideologies were supported by social practices in the major institutions of the modern patriarchal capitalist society (Hanmer, 1978; Dworkin, 1981; MacKinnon, 1982; Frye, 1983). In doing this the radical feminist anti-violence movement demonstrated the role of male power in the legitimation of violence and the inextricable links between power and violence.

Within feminism, dissent and debate was constant throughout the 1970s and radical feminist views were often contested as different and often competing explanations and solutions to male dominance and violence were posited. One of the main criticisms of second wave feminist explanations of violence was the tendency to homogenize experiences and therefore to erase difference (Williams, 1996). The suppression of difference, through the constitution of a universalizing narrative of women's oppression, the coherent category 'woman' and the claim that all women should put the women's revolution first, alienated black, colonized and third world women (O'Shane 1976; hooks, 1981; Moraga and Anzaldua, 1983; Mohanty, 1988). It was amid these bitter contestations about race, class and sexuality that both lesbian and cultural feminism emerged in the mid-1970s.

Cultural feminism stressed the spiritual and moved away from explicitly political activities (Gould Davis, 1972; Burris, 1973; Bunch, 1975) and similar to early radical feminism, it was based on essentialist notions of sexual difference, with men and women being ascribed fixed and universal characteristics determined by biology, nature or psychology. However, rather than constituting women as being disadvantaged because of these differences, this was reversed with women's biology now seen as an advantage, and their maternal qualities critical to the development of an alternate women's culture. Discourses of women as essentially peaceful and non-violent began to emerge (Johnston, 1974; Morgan, 1978). Cultural feminists claimed that women were different and superior to men with lesbian cultural feminists extending this argument and claiming lesbians were superior to heterosexual women (Allegro, 1975).

This coincided with some radical feminists challenging the heterosexual experience as that of all women (see for example Summers, 1975). Lesbians who were radical feminists began to resist what they considered as totalizing definitions of radical feminism and began to generate different explanations. Radical lesbian feminism emerged and located itself at the intersection of radical feminism and gay liberation (Williams, 1996). While gender was seen as the primary determiner of oppression, heterosexuality was constituted as the main form of male domination. Women, it was argued, were unable to be free of patriarchal control as long as they remained involved with men. This reinforced heterosexuality as a natural and superior form of sexuality while simultaneously working to oppress lesbians and gay men (Bunch, 1975). Early radical lesbian feminists used the argument that patriarchal order is secured through compulsory heterosexuality and the suppression of lesbianism, claiming that lesbianism was a political position, not just a sexual preference (see for example CLIT Collective, 1974; Brown, 1976). All women, it was argued, have the potential to be lesbians, the only limitation to this being the dominance of patriarchal culture (Johnston, 1974). Separatism was generated as some radical lesbian feminists extended this argument by proclaiming that *all* feminists must take a political stance, renounce their hetero-sexual privilege and purposefully and consciously choose to intentionally posi-tion themselves as political lesbians with a primary emotional commitment and affiliation to women (Bunch, 1975; Brown, 1976). Lesbianism challenged patri-archal practices representing a model of egalitarian relationships between equals and the possibility of a life determined by women for their own and other women's benefits (Brown, 1976). Radical lesbian feminists were depicted as active, autonomous, self-determining, independent and responsible people already equal to men (Gutter Dyke Collective, 1988). Both cultural and radical lesbian feminism saw other feminists as anti-feminist, and diminished, de-legitimized and devalued the part played by radical feminists who were heterosexual in eradicating patriarchy (Johnston, 1974; English, Hollibaugh and Rubin, 1982; Echols, 1989).

In doing this, radical and cultural lesbian feminists constituted themselves as a privileged form of feminism that was well positioned to overthrow patriarchy. Values of egalitarianism, non-violence and non-hierarchical practices replaced the dominant values of patriarchy that had shaped and limited women's lives, generat-ing discourses of lesbian utopia as lesbians were seen as peace loving, nurturant and non-competitive, with intimate lesbian relationships idealized. As lesbian separatist communities emerged these values became the basis for the 'ideal' community. They were also a powerful influence for many lesbians who were actively involved in fighting for and developing services for women, such as rape crisis, domestic vio-lence, and emergency accommodation with many women's services often modelled on these values. While bitter recriminations in the women's movement, inflamed by the sex wars over pornography, sadomasochism and butch/femme roles led to dis-agreements over the notion of a lesbian utopia, the discursive constitution of lesbian relationships as non-violent has remained a powerful influence, playing a part in masking intimate partner violence between lesbians.

These powerful discourses of lesbians as loving, egalitarian and non-competitive, effectively closed the space for any discussion of the possibility of violence in lesbian intimate relationships, resulting in denial of its existence. This coupled with the theorizing of violence which focused on male violence against women (which is hardly surprising in the context of tackling patriarchal oppression and given the extent of male violence against women) has further constrained our knowledge and understandings about intimate partner violence between lesbians, reinforcing both the heteronormative conceptualization of domestic violence and the invisibility and silencing of this violence. This invisibility has been chal-lenged more recently by an increasing literature on domestic violence in lesbian relationships which has helped acknowledge that this violence does exist. It has also directly contributed to theorizing intimate partner violence between lesbians.

Theorizing intimate partner violence between lesbians

Since 1986 when the first book on intimate partner violence between lesbians was published, literature and research on intimate partner violence has emerged from countries in the Western World (see, for example Ristock, 2002; Renzetti, 1992; Kaschak, 2001). The literature broadly falls into three main areas: establishing the extent of intimate partner violence between lesbians; explaining or theorizing intimate partner violence between lesbians and exploring lesbians' experiences of intimate partner violence (Irwin, 2007, in press). While the exploration of lesbians' experiences of domestic violence and establishing the extent of domestic violence in lesbian relationships have both been an important aspect of legitimating the issue, it is the debates around the theorizing of intimate partner violence between lesbians I will now briefly overview.

Controversy has raged mainly around the role gender plays in explaining or theorizing intimate partner violence between lesbians. There have been two main approaches. One approach explores the similarities in intimate partner violence in same-sex relationships, that is comparisons between lesbians and gay men (for example, Dutton, 1994; Island and Letellier, 1991). This approach tends to focus on either psychological (Dutton, 1994; Island and Letellier, 1991) or socio-psychological theories (Merrill, 1996). Those who focus on psychological theories often define gender as biological and dismiss feminist gender based explanations of domestic violence, claiming that the existence of violence in gay male and lesbian relationships shows that gender is not relevant (Dutton, 1994; Island and Letellier, 1991). Those who draw on socio-psychological theories are more likely to acknowledge the complexities of intimate partner violence in same-sex relationships, taking into account social issues such as how homophobia can influence experiences (Merrill, 1996).

The other approach focuses on violence in lesbian relationships comparing intimate partner violence between lesbians and heterosexual women rather than the gender blended category of same-sex. It draws on radical feminist theories conceptualizing domestic violence between lesbians as a function of gender based oppression (see, for example, Eaton, 1994). More recently explanations based primarily on gender have been critiqued for being heterocentric and treating all women the same, excluding particular women whose experience may be different because of their situational locations of race, class and sexual identity (Girshick, 1996; Kaye/Kantrowitz, 1992; Renzetti, 1999; Ristock, 2002; McClennen, 2005). It is argued that these structural and contextual influences shape experiences and in order to make sense of the specificities of violence in lesbian relationships, it is necessary to unpack and explore how gender and other differences can produce lesbians' experiences of violence (Kaye/Kantrowitz, 1992: 37).

I have argued that dominant discourses around domestic violence have both limited and shaped the ways we theorize and understand violence against lesbians. As social practices these have influenced the ways lesbians understand and talk about domestic violence in their relationships, contributing to both the invisibility and silence around this violence. This has meant that naming and responding to this violence has been difficult as there has not been the language nor the conceptual understandings to do so. The normative discourses of domestic violence as a heterosexual issue have helped to sustain this invisibility and contributed to the heteronormative responses to this violence. However, as lesbian's stories of intimate partner violence have begun to circulate we are beginning to understand how the discourses around domestic violence and lesbian utopia impact on the material worlds of lesbians and develop more nuanced understandings of the specificities and complexities of violence in these women's lives. It is lesbians' stories of domestic violence to which I now turn to illustrate my argument.

Stories of intimate partner violence in lesbian relationships

The stories I draw on were collected in research I undertook in Australia with lesbians who identified as having lived with violence in a lesbian relationship. I interviewed twenty-one lesbians exploring how understandings of intimate partner violence between lesbians are constituted and how these influenced, shaped and produced lesbians' experiences of intimate partner violence. The participants came from diverse backgrounds. The majority of women were white Australians with the minority being Aboriginal Australians or born in overseas countries. For almost all their first language was English. Some women had tertiary education qualifications; others had not completed high school. Almost all were employed, but some were receiving some form of government income support. A wide variety of occupations were represented including nurses, community and social workers, teachers, marketing executives, beauty consultants, solicitors and security guards. Almost all of the participants recounted how it took some time for them to acknowledge the violence and how the decision to leave was often a long and painful process. The abuse included combinations of physical, emotional, sexual, economic and/or social abuse. The denial, silence and invisibility of violence in lesbian relationships impacted on the women's experiences in a number of ways. This included their struggles to name the violence and their encounters with the police and counsellors.

Naming the violence

Naming violence is a political act and has been a critical feature of feminist activism. However, limited language and understanding and the lack of talk about intimate partner violence between lesbians has contributed to the difficulty in speaking out just as it did for women and girls who courageously spoke out about male violence in the 1970s. Many of the women interviewed did not recognize what was happening to them as they thought of domestic violence as a heterosexual issue that did not apply to lesbians. Betty was one of these:

> And there was never anything out there that even hinted about lesbian domestic violence. And I just think, if there was something – something. 'cause it was all so heterosexual. And – even the words 'lesbian domestic violence'. Like 'domestic violence' is based very much on a heterosexual

concept. But, I think it's been really, really good to be able to use it. For something that is just so hard to sort of like label. And I think it's important to label it. When it's not sort of discussed. (Betty)

Isabella who had been on a committee at a women's refuge also struggled to name the violence as she saw domestic violence as a heterosexual issue. She had recognized that there were problems in her relationship but did not see this as domestic violence. She experienced emotional, social and economic abuse and although she was never physically abused her partner destroyed furniture and threatened her.

> I didn't frame it as domestic violence. And I just thought, being a lesbian, it's really difficult. People aren't going to believe me. I've been a chairperson at a women's refuge for about five years. It's just so ironic. And I never ever saw the domestic violence as domestic violence. (Isabella)

Some of the women were unable to name the abuse while they were in the relationship. Carmel, a forty-year-old teacher, experienced physical and emotional, economic abuse. It was only after she left the relationship that she could name the abuse but at the same time she began questioning her silence and inaction, seeing herself as somehow complicit and taking some of the responsibility. Dominant discourses of femininity constituting women as nurturing, caring and responsible for relationships and their success (or failure) can play a critical part in shaping responses.

> She was wrapping me up from the beginning, and then organizing things that I didn't realize, the implications for. You know what I mean? It was just incredible. Like, I knew – you know how you know something, but you're not labelling it, or putting a name to it? Or really trying to bring it to your conscious forethought, because you know if you do, you'll have to do something about it. (Carmel)

Aileen did not experience physical abuse and was unsure about what was happening but did not label it as violence.

> I didn't know what was going on. I didn't know how to deal with it. 'Cause I didn't know what it was. It's only been very recently that I've been able to go back and start to frame some of it. (Aileen)

Later in the interview Aileen indicated that she understood what was going on, but was unable to label it as violence. Commenting that she was really 'hooked into it' she, like Carmel was honing in on her responsibility for, and complicity in the violence.

And I knew it was happening, but I still – I wasn't calling it abusive. Yeah, I was certainly hooked into it. Real easy. And I sort of alternate between thinking, 'Well, maybe it wasn't abusive. If I'm not able to use that language, maybe it wasn't'. But then, when I tell incidents, other people say, 'Well, that's dreadful, you know. That was really abusive.' (Aileen)

Several of the women commented they did not believe women could abuse. One of these women, Shirley believed that women are not violent so did not see coercive sex as abuse.

She was drinking still, and her abuse was getting worse, and she – she was being more forceful, especially in terms of sex. And I'd say that I experienced rape on a couple of occasions. And all the time I can't believe this is happening. Women don't do this. She'd keep me up till two and three in the morning, wanting sex, abusing me, me trying to extricate myself. (Shirley)

It is only when we create the space for lesbians to speak out and be heard about their experiences of intimate partner violence that we will begin to develop more nuanced understandings about the violence and develop appropriate responses.

Seeking support

Support has been identified as critical in recovering from violence, often acting as a buffer to counter the negative consequences of the violence (Carlson, McNutt, Choi and Rose, 2002). However, in order to seek support women have to expose the violence and be confident of being heard and believed (Dobash and Dobash, 1992; Mullender and Morley, 1994). This can raise particular issues for lesbians because it means they have to deal with both the exposure of their sexuality, as well as exposure of the violence. Decisions about seeking support are influenced by a complex array of factors often related to whether a request for assistance is likely to result in a positive outcome. For some women this exposure is beyond their control as neighbours or onlookers report incidents of physical violence to the police, or the women seek medical attention following severe physical abuse. In this study many of the women's experiences of seeking support were dominated by heteronormative assumptions from mainstream service providers. These assumptions framed and produced limited understandings of the way lesbians interact, shaping how service providers responded. The women in the study had contact with an array of service providers including counsellors, police, medical services, emergency housing and other support services. In this chapter I focus on the women's engagement with police and counsellors.

Police

While some of the women who participated in this research had contact with the police, for most this was not a choice they actively made, as neighbours, friends or family were often the initiators of this contact. For particular groups ambivalent attitudes towards police involvement can be magnified by previous negative experiences. For example, stories have circulated about police mistreatment of gay men and lesbians which can influence attitudes and beliefs that the police may act in discriminatory ways or not act at all. These play a part in shaping decisions about whether to seek police assistance. Themes to emerge from the women's engagement with the police were the difficulty the police had in recognizing domestic violence between lesbians, the trivialization of such violence and the tendency to transpose heteronormative understandings of domestic violence.

Several of the women commented that they had not considered going to the police because they feared they would not be believed or that the police would take no action because they were lesbians. Ruth had several contacts with the police. Her own experiences led her to believe that the police discounted and trivialized domestic violence between lesbians:

> They probably – seeing two girls – they probably think 'Those two dykes, fighting again' – they'd been up here a few times. (Ruth)

Margaret recounted how she and a friend went to the police with an array of evidence from extremely vicious physical abuse which had been attended by police at the time.

> And he told us that these matters were not a matter for the police – that the police – the good police – were very busy dealing with real life crime, and it was a whole waste of the police officers' time. They'd been with us for at least over an hour – and wasting their time. (Margaret)

Margaret pursued this at another police station and her ex-partner was subsequently convicted of assault.

Some of the stories recounted by the women about their engagement with police and other service providers illustrated that often when there is limited understanding about intimate partner violence that practitioners often impose a normative heterosexual model of domestic violence to lesbians which can lead to inappropriate responses. For many practitioners, including the police, the need to identify a perpetrator and a victim is important but in situations of intimate partner violence between lesbians, the absence of a gender marker, as there is in heterosexual domestic violence, can pose problems. Frequently, understandings of heterosexual domestic violence are transposed to lesbian domestic violence but they don't always fit neatly, as Sharon's quote demonstrates:

> The police – the guy said to me 'listen mate. The thing is we've got to stop treating it like lesbians are different. The thing is, there's the bloke and there's the woman. And you're the bloke and she's the woman.' (Sharon)

Responses such as this can be prompted by heteronormative assumptions, producing heterosexist or homophobic reactions which can deter lesbians from seeking help, leaving them isolated and compromising their safety.

Counsellors

The women in this study were more likely to seek assistance from counsellors than any other formal supports. Negative responses from counsellors play an integral part in influencing women not to seek further assistance and also contribute to the invisibility of the violence. Positive responses can be experienced as empowering and can support women to make changes in their lives. Angela began to believe her relationship was abusive and she and her partner sought counselling. Her experience, however, made it more difficult for her to recognize the violence and discouraged her from seeking further support.

> And when we went to counselling, I realized there was no place for me in the room, and that I would really rather just walk out, get in the car and drive home. The counsellor didn't seem to me at all to think it was in any way abusive. In fact, I felt a bit to blame in the counsellor's eyes. Like I – and I think I felt weak. (Angela)

Isabella sought help from a counsellor but despite the indicators of violence, these were not recognized by the counsellor.

> But, the other thing was that I did attempt to do something about our relationship. I went to counselling, with her, to a psychologist. But the psychologist I think, at that time – I don't think – I think she just didn't understand about lesbian relationships. And I don't think she could see that it was – I think if she'd been able to frame it as domestic violence. (Isabella)

The limited knowledge and skills counsellors have in working with lesbians was a recurring theme. Some lesbians experienced this as indicating homophobic or heterosexist assumptions, attitudes and beliefs, while others saw it as a limited awareness of the issues that lesbians confront in their daily lives. Whatever the reason it signifies that lack of awareness of the issues that lesbians confront in their daily lives, and of domestic violence as a possibility in lesbian relationships, can limit counsellors' responses to lesbians seeking help, reinforcing the invisibility of domestic violence.

Implications for human service professionals

Practitioners and policy makers in the human, health and community services face a number of challenges in tackling the invisibility and the consequent heteronormative assumptions that underlie responses to intimate partner violence between lesbians.

Much of the service provision is underpinned by heteronormative assumptions and the challenge is to increase awareness of violence in lesbian relationships in ways that do not further increase discrimination against lesbians or the lesbian community, and do not detract from the extent of male violence against women. Mainstream agencies, both government and non-government, need to take responsibility in educating their employees about the existence of domestic violence between lesbians, as well as ensuring their services are both accessible and relevant to lesbians. Tertiary education institutions who educate/train health, human and community service providers have a similar responsibility.

The development of tertiary, secondary and preventive services that are safe and relevant is critical. To enable women to make more informed choices about the services they use, organizations could be encouraged to be explicit about the philosophical basis that underpins their work. Within services there is also a need to question heteronormative assumptions that pervade much of the existing service delivery. If mainstream agencies are to be available to all women, they need to examine who has access to their services and who does not. The subsequent development of programmes to address these gaps in services is vital. Similar to heterosexual women, lesbians who experience domestic violence need to be able to access a variety of different services. These could include counselling, court support and group programmes. It is crucial that service providers have knowledge and understanding of both the variety of ways in which lesbians experience violence and the issues that they have to deal with in their lives which may impact upon this. Agencies have responsibility to provide ongoing training and supervision for their staff to ensure the relevance of their services for lesbians.

While social policies in more recent years have attempted to accommodate diversity in relation to domestic violence in general, they are informed by understandings of women (and men) that work to obscure the specificities of some groups' needs and interests. Lesbians are one such group whose particular interests are rarely dealt with explicitly. Policy responses have generally been based on heteronormative assumptions, not accommodating the different and often heterosexist contexts in which abuse occurs. The challenge is to encourage and provide information to policy makers so they can develop policy that accurately reflects and takes into account the concerns of lesbians and their particular needs and interests.

There is a need for much more in-depth knowledge about the complexities of violence in lesbian relationships, particularly how the personal, social and political contexts influence how women experience violence in their lives. The need for continued research in this area is evident.

Political activity, as always, remains crucial to achieving positive changes in the lives of women. One of the most important ways forward, underpinning all these challenges, is ongoing exposure of heterosexism and its consequences, and fighting for lesbians' social acceptance. Continuing to fight for accessible and relevant services for lesbians should remain a priority.

Chapter summary

**Challenging the second closet: intimate
partner violence between lesbians**

- In this chapter it is argued that early feminist theorizing of domestic violence, premised on male violence against women, has become the basis for
  normative understandings of domestic violence which have unintentionally worked to make abuse in intimate lesbian relationships invisible.
- This invisibility has been further exacerbated by theoretical approaches
  which have constituted lesbians as privileged subjects, producing discourses
  of lesbian utopia which have idealized intimate lesbian relationships.
- The argument is illustrated using research undertaken in Australia which
  explored lesbian's experiences of domestic violence.
- The women's stories showed that irrespective of the generation of recent
  literature challenging the early homogenizing explanations of domestic
  violence and positing more nuanced understandings, these normative discourses of domestic violence with their heteronormative assumptions have
  played a powerful role in influencing how the lesbians make sense of, and
  responded to, the abuse in their relationships.
- Many of the women in this study initially remained silent about their abuse
  because they saw domestic violence as a heterosexual issue which did not
  affect them.
- Some women struggled to identify the violence because they believed that
  this did not happen in lesbian relationships. Others could not believe a
  woman could be violent.
- The prevalent message that domestic violence does not exist in lesbian
  relationships often meant there was no language to describe what the
  women were experiencing.
- However, despite the lack of language to articulate the violence it still had
  a huge impact on their lives.
- These dominant discourses have also shaped and limited responses to intimate partner violence between lesbians from service providers in the
  health, human and community services.

9 Violence against women in rural settings

Margot Rawsthorne

This chapter explores violence against women in rural settings. It argues that violence against women in rural settings is enabled by oppressive social norms and relations. These social norms shape intimate relationships in ways that make women vulnerable to violence. They include rigid gender roles and the privatization and tolerance of violence. Contrary to stereotypical images of rural communities, the nature of social relations in rural communities has increased women's vulnerability to violence. Multiple bonded ties create barriers to women gaining or seeking support to escape violence. This chapter adopts Lori Heise's ecological framework (1998; Heise, Ellsberg and Gottmoeller, 2002), conceptualizing violence against women 'as a multifaceted phenomenon grounded in an interplay among personal, situational, and socio-cultural factors' (1998: 263–4). Not only does this interplay cause violence against women in rural settings it also perpetuates the silence and inadequate response to this violence. Violence against women in many rural settings is still condoned, despite over thirty years of feminist activism. Whilst this chapter adopts Heise's ecological framework it needs to be acknowledged that there are other ways of understanding violence against women which are explored in Barbara Fawcett's chapter and in Jude Irwin's chapter.

In order to adopt an international perspective, three very different countries have been chosen to profile rural women's experiences. These are Australia, Uganda and Bangladesh. These countries have been chosen to highlight both the commonality and heterogeneity of women's experiences and the importance of context. However, prior to profiling the experiences of rural women in these three countries and drawing from the research evidence, a number of conceptual issues require clarification. First, what is understood by the concept 'rural'? Second, what do we know about the concept of 'community' in rural settings? Finally, how do we explain violence against rural women? This chapter will explore these issues and will conclude with a brief discussion of the challenges facing human service professionals in preventing violence against rural women.

Throughout this chapter the terms 'violence against women' will be used to acknowledge the dominant experience of women as victims of interpersonal violence. This is not to imply that males are not also victims of violence. In profiling the experiences of rural women in different countries the indigenous term for that cultural setting will be employed, for example 'wife bashing' in the Ugandan context.

Conceptual issues

Rural settings

To focus on the experiences of rural women requires firstly some discussion of what we mean by 'rural'. Within sociology the concept of 'rural' is strongly contested, with significant debate since the 1970s about the meaning of the concept (Hart, Larson and Lishner, 2005). Population density has commonly been used as a proxy for 'rural'. The Organization of Economic Co-operation and Development (OECD), for example, define any areas with a population density of less than 150 inhabitants per square kilometre as rural (Ocana-Riola and Sanchez-Cantalejo, 2005). Critics of this approach point out that there is no accepted population figure and definitions vary both between countries and within countries. A population approach also fails to consider the social or cultural context.

In more recent years we have seen a move away from population or land-use definitions to a recognition that 'rural' is a 'multifaceted concept about which there is no universal agreement' (Hart *et al.*, 2005) making it a 'slippery signifier' (Share, 1997: 2). This lack of agreement creates challenges for researchers seeking greater methodological rigour in relation to definitional issues (Hart *et al.*, 2005; Ocana-Riola and Sanchez-Cantalejo, 2005). When using the concept 'rural' researchers include: land-use (agricultural or extractive activities); geography (pastoral landscapes); demographic structures (ageing population with out-migration of post-school young people); low population density; and distinct socio-cultural milieus (in the Australian context, cultural events like the Debutante Ball and the Bachelors' and Spinsters' Balls). Additionally, the urbanization of many traditionally rural areas suggest that settlement viewed as a continuum from high density urban to sparsely settled remoteness may be more useful than an urban/rural dichotomy (Ocana-Riola and Sanchez-Cantalejo, 2005).

> [R]ural areas are not distinguished from urban areas only according to the inhabitants forming the core population, but also through variables reflecting their economic, health, social and cultural circumstances. As a result, rural and urban would be the two opposite ends of a continuum that describes the geographic areas in a region or country.
>
> (Ocana-Riola and Sanchez-Cantalejo, 2005: 249)

Understanding women's experiences as shaped by a continuum of settlement patterns rather than a binary categorization alerts us to the commonality and heterogeneity of women's experiences. Within popular and academic culture 'rural' has often taken on an 'other' ('non-urban') status, implicitly oppositional or binary in nature. This approach suggests a 'uniform' rural experience, failing to recognize the enormous diversity in experiences within nations and globally. Rural women's experiences will be shaped by the specific history, economic, political, social and cultural context in which they experience violence.

Both the social context and social model framing each geographical area must be taken into account. History, tradition, idiosyncrasies and social circumstances of each region mean that the area has particular features that are not necessarily identical to those seen in areas in other regions. As a result, the determinants of rurality may differ between countries with distinct social settings.

(Ocana-Riola and Sanchez-Cantalejo, 2005: 249)

Community in rural settings

Like the concept of 'rural', the concept of 'community' is contested, complex and shifting. It also has a long tradition of debate and discussion in the academic literature. Two contrasting approaches to understanding 'community' are currently evident in the literature: abandonment (by postmodern and globalization critics) and engagement (by social capital theorists). What this highlights is the importance of adopting a critical perspective in thinking about 'community'. The meaning given to 'community' is shaped socially, politically and historically. Individuals will understand 'community' in different ways in different settings and at difference times. The concept of 'community' can be based on geographic location or place, on identity or a common or shared interest and a 'sense of belonging' (Cohen, 1985; Dempsey, 1992).

The concept of community in rural settings has, particularly in western countries, been subject to romanticized, emotive language. Culturally many highly urbanized countries hark-back to a romanticized past in which 'everyone knew everyone' and there was a 'real' sense of community (Frank, 2003).

> [C]ommunity … is the kind of world which is not, regrettably, available to us – but which we would dearly love to inhabit and which we hope to repossess.
>
> (Bauman, 2001: 3)

This rural idyllic mythology renders invisible the divisions of power, privilege, disempowerment and deprivation present within all communities (Schulman and Anderson, 1999; Pugh, 2003; Shortall, 2004). Frank, exploring the role of the media in shaping understandings of rural communities in the United States, revealed the recurrence of certain motifs indicative of core cultural values. Central motifs included: residents all know each other; the town is 'sleepy'; people leave their doors unlocked and their keys in their cars; and terrible things are not supposed to happen in 'good places' (rural communities) (Frank, 2003: 211). Drawing on the work of Tönnies (1957) many commentators attribute *Gemeinschaft* qualities to rural communities: personal and enduring; intimate; involving a person in his or her totality; trustworthy and honest; and loyal to friends and to the community (Dempsey, 1992: 32–3). The imagery of rural communities creates meaning not only for those 'outsiders' but also for 'insiders'.

Social relations for some in rural settings does indeed mirror the rural idyllic. The proximity of life, shared social norms and multiple social ties can lead to a life rich in social capital. Rural communities can be characterized by supportive networks, reciprocity, trust, shared norms and a sense of social agency (Onyx and Bullen, 2000). Empirical research, however, alerts us to risks inherent in communities with a dominance of bonded social capital. Different types of social capital are required to bridge and link communities with others. Communities with strong social ties tend to be inward-looking and do not always enhance social cohesion. They have the capacity to protect paternalism, sexism and racism by maintaining existing power structures and excluding people outside the mainstream from work and community (Wallis and Dollery, 2002; Mendes, 2004).

Whilst acknowledging its complexity, this chapter argues that the concept of community remains important in understanding rural women's experience of violence. The next section discusses how social norms and social relations can hide or deny violence against women in rural settings as well as shaping women's access to support services.

Violence against women in rural settings

Awareness and policy action relating to violence against women varies internationally. Whilst organizations such as the World Health Organization and the United Nations have recognized the global scale of violence against women there remain considerable differences in community awareness and government action across the world. In first world countries, awareness and policy action relating to the experiences of rural women occurred earlier than in developing countries. There is, however, increasing evidence and awareness of the 'magnitude of the problem of domestic violence in developing countries' (Koenig, Lutalo, Zhao, et al., 2003: 53).

In 2002 the World Health Organization produced the first World Report on Violence and Health. This Report found unacceptable levels of violence, particularly perpetrated against women and children. Naved and Lars argue:

> Violence against women is a worldwide problem, transcending cultural, geographic, religious, social and economic boundaries. ... A consensus is emerging that personal, economic, social and cultural factors combine to cause abuse.
>
> (Naved and Lars, 2005: 289)

Adopting an ecological framework, these factors combine within 'embedded levels of causality' (Heise, 1998: 264). This framework enables the individual(s), their context and broader socio-cultural factors to be considered. The ecological framework explains gender-based violence as arising from the 'interplay of personal, situational, and sociocultural factors' (Heise *et al.*, 2002: S7). Four concentric circles are used to represent: individual personal histories; the immediate social context in which the abuse takes place (microsystem); the formal and informal institutions and social structures (exosystem); and finally the general cultural views and attitudes (macrosystem). The framework provides a way of conceptualizing the complex interplay of factors that contribute to violence against women but should not be viewed as static, linear or categorical. In thinking about the processes that shape women's experiences we need to be aware of the interdependencies of the layers or concentric circles. Individual behaviours are shaped by social norms.

The personal histories and microsystems in which rural women experience violence is likely to have much in common with women living in other settings. It is argued, however, that the experience of rural women is strongly influenced by what could be conceived as the 'outer rings' of an ecological framework: the exosystem and macrosystem factors (Heise, 1998; Heise *et al.*, 2002). The third ring or the exosystem highlights that: '[a]t the community level women's isolation and lack of social support, together with male peer groups that condone and legitimize men's violence, predict higher rates of violence' (Heise *et al.*, 2002: S8).

Rural women are vulnerable to isolation and a lack of social support. This isolation can result from distance, but also from a deliberate strategy of the perpetrator of violence to reduce women's relationships and networks. In many rural settings around the world communication technology such as the telephone are limited. This can occur even in western countries such as Australia where 'bush' women travel extended distances in order to access phones. In addition to telecommunication, transport and the low likelihood of future work (and hence independence) also acted as barriers to leaving violent situations for Kentucky women (Websdale, 1995). In more developing countries, this technology may not be available at all. Many of the social support systems (both formal and informal) are not available in rural settings. Police and emergency services may be located at a distance, refuges or shelters are fewer, counselling and other professional assistance more limited (Bosch and Schumm, 2004). Women's ability to re-establish themselves after leaving a violent relationship is also hindered by the lack of housing and employment options. Access to support services is consistently identified in research as a major impediment to women leaving violent relationships (Jategaonkar, Greaves, Poole, McCullough and Chabot, 2005; Van Hightower and Gorton, 2002).

Poor social infrastructure is exacerbated by social practices that place the blame for violence on victims. Victim blaming myths influence service provision to women in rural settings throughout the world. Women are seen as 'deserving' and responsible for violence through their actions or inactions. How cultural myths enable violence against women is highlighted by research in Zimbabwe (Hindin, 2003), South Africa (Kim and Motsei, 2002) and India (Jejeebhoy, 1998). These myths are concrete expressions of condoning and legitimizing male violence against women and often have widespread community support. Van Hightower and Gorton argue that without adequate service delivery, responses to violence against women in rural settings will continue without change to the 'socio-political ethos that supports victim blaming' (2002: 870).

Violence against women is supported by exosystem beliefs that view husband and wife relations as being outside of public scrutiny, a potential outcome of strongly bonded communities with poor bridging social capital which is characteristic of some rural settings (Onyx and Bullen, 2000). The 'closeness' of rural communities contributes to the hidden nature of violence against women. Dempsey (2002a) argues women who seek support, or who leave their violent partners, risk censure through gossip or ostracism for failing to keep family matters private, or failing to keep the family unit intact. In her study of the experiences of Canadian women, Hornosty (1995) highlights the role of religion in supporting very traditional patriarchal gender behaviours.

Cultural myths surrounding 'good places' enable the public silencing of women's experience of interpersonal violence. Studies in the United States and Australia suggest that the network of relationships in rural communities creates a barrier for police dealing with domestic violence (Websdale, 1995; Coorey, 1990). Barriers to adequate service responses are also evident in other forms of abuse such as adolescent sexual assault in rural settings (Rawsthorne, 2003). As mentioned previously, rural communities are characterized by bonded social capital in which people have multiple strong social ties to others. 'Naming' violence in rural settings breaches the community's understanding of itself and stereotyped portrayals of 'safety'. Additionally, formal support provided by the police, health, schools or other agencies are influenced by cultural norms that silence women's experiences of violence. Previous research has highlighted the patriarchal or conservative attitudes of key supports for rural women in western countries: the clergy (Hornosty, 1995), doctors (Bagshaw, Chung, Couch, Lilburn and Wadhan, 2000) and police (Coorey, 1990). Discussing the experiences of battered women in Texas, Van Hightower and Gorton note that 'policies in rural areas tend to be shaped by institutionalised patriarchal values' (2002: 869).

The silence that surrounds violence against women in rural settings may be interpreted by violent males as tacit support. The lack of intervention, either by informal or formal systems, can be viewed by violent men as support (Hearn, 1998; Bagshaw et al., 2000; Dobash and Dobash, 1998).

The fourth ring or macrosystem factors appear also at play in rural settings. Heise and colleagues argue:

> At the society level studies around the world have found that violence against women is most common where gender roles are rigidly defined and enforced and where the concept of masculinity is linked to toughness, male honor, or dominance. Other cultural norms associated with abuse include tolerance of physical punishment of women and children, acceptance of violence as a means to settle interpersonal disputes, and the perception that men have 'ownership' of women.
>
> (Heise et al., 2002: S8)

Researchers exploring gender relations in rural communities often conclude that patriarchal structures and attitudes remain embedded in rural culture. Gender roles are often rigidly defined and enforced through violence (Alston, 1997; Campbell and Phillips, 1997). Male breadwinner/female home-carer remain the dominant gender roles in many rural settings, although this construction hides the extent of outside work many rural women undertake. Discussing rural New Zealand and Australia, Campbell and Phillips argue that there has been a 'conspicuous gap' in the research about rural men. Drawing on Hearn (1992) they note that '[b]y failing to make a distinction between the normative male subject and the specific nature of masculine social practice the existence of such practices are effectively shielded from any sustained analysis' (Campbell and Phillips, 1997: 107).

Rural masculinity is strongly tied to hegemonic masculinity in which maleness is equated to dominance over others, particularly women (Carrigan, Connell and Lee, 1987; Connell, 2000). Hegemonic masculinity is supported by both men and women through ideology and practice that reacts against counter-definitions of gender. Exploring sites of gender practice (such as the pub, sporting clubs and the bachelor and spinster ball) Campbell and Phillips conclude that 'the structure of social interaction within rural society is aggressively masculine' (1997: 123).

> This rural hegemonic masculinity encompasses a range of manifestations all of which have the basic ingredients of the creation of a symbolically masculine world, patterns of male interaction that both create and reinforce masculine hegemony through the use of norms and solidarity, and the total rejection of any form of domestic or feminine control.
>
> (Campbell and Phillips, 1997: 123)

Profiles of rural women's experience of violence

Australia

> … they do get you out in the never never where you have no contact with anybody and they are the only one in your life and I don't think people realize you know that that is very important for them to do that. They've got the wife there and there is nothing she can do and it's not a matter of picking up the phone and somebody coming to pick you up, it just doesn't happen.
>
> (Chantelle quoted in Trickett, 2006: 67–8)

Australia is an affluent western country that is highly urbanized despite being a vast continent. The country's population (20 million) is concentrated on the eastern seaboard with large settlements stretching from Melbourne to Brisbane. The continent's geography and human settlement patterns has shaped Australian culture. Rural communities ('over the divide') are seen as different from the way most Australians live. Rural people are strongly stereotyped and rural myths have been cultivated to signify what is deemed quintessentially 'Australian' – hard working pioneers, struggle against the elements with the support of 'mates'. Women's contribution to the development of rural Australia is often overlooked with 'farmer' still understood as masculine (Alston, 1995). Prominent Australian studies point to the cultural dominance of men in their titles, including 'A Man's Town' (Dempsey, 1992) and 'The Good Old Rule' (Poiner, 1990).

In this context, government policies fail to recognize the extent of violence in rural communities, despite statistical evidence, and the phenomenon is predominantly hidden. The exception is when the violence involves Indigenous communities, when it becomes an issue of high media interest. An undercurrent of racism – pathologizing Indigenous culture – then becomes evident. Violence against and within Indigenous communities requires urgent attention and is discussed in-depth in Chapter 5.

More generally, violence in rural communities within Australia is unacceptably high. Given the hidden nature of violence against women in rural settings and the many barriers to receiving support, these reported cases are also likely to be only a small proportion of the overall problem. The NSW Bureau of Crime Statistics and Research (2005) provides detailed data on apprehended violence orders, domestic violence related assault and sexual assault for the most populous state in Australia. Table 9.1 highlights that some rural regions have considerably higher levels of recorded criminal incidents than the Sydney Statistical Division. These regions are generally remote, sparsely populated and poorly serviced. Drawing on the ecological framework, explanations for the discrepancies in recorded criminal incidents must go beyond the individual personalities involved or the dynamics within a specific relationship. For women in Far Western New South Wales to be more than four times more vulnerable to sexual assault than women in Sydney requires other explanations.

Patriarchal values that legitimize or deny violence against women often inform key institutions in the third circle or exosystem. Both the formal and informal systems in rural settings fail to support women experiencing violence, tending instead to hold her responsible (Coorey, 1990; Alston, 1997; Rawsthorne, 2003). This is evident in Aretha's experience of seeking police intervention in a small rural town in South Australia: distance was not a factor as she lived close by the Police station:

> … I could've been lying bleeding on the floor for that time [police response] … they were hoping that the situation would diffuse before they got there and that is exactly what had happened but it may not have been the case
>
> (quoted in Trickett, 2006: 63)

These values were also evident in schools, among doctors, health workers and community workers in relation to young rural women's experience of sexual violence (Rawsthorne, 2003). Strong relationship ties (or bonded social capital) in rural settings act to impede support from both informal and formal systems. 'Everyone knowing everyone' creates a barrier to seeking assistance with confidentiality. Family reputations often determine how a claim of violence is received and the support offered (Macklin, 1997; Rawsthorne, 2003).

Table 9.1 Recorded criminal incidents, 2003 to 2005: Statistical Division

Statistical Division where offence occurred	Assault – domestic violence related		Sexual assault	
	Number	Rate per 100,000 population	Number	Rate per 100,000 population
Sydney	13,658	322.7	1,889	44.6
Far West	261	1,101.9	34	143.5
North Western	1,268	1,067.9	169	142.3
Northern	1,013	565.5	194	108.3
Murrumbidgee	713	465.5	115	75.1
NSW (State)	25,870	384.3	4,016	59.7

Source: NSW Bureau of Crime Statistics and Research (2005)

Uganda

Uganda is a landlocked country in the East African region and has been plagued by violent conflict for much of its history since gaining independence from the British in the 1960s. Uganda is home to many different ethnic groups, none of whom forms a majority of the population. Around forty different languages are regularly and currently in use in the country. English became the official language of Uganda after independence. Eighty-five per cent of the population is Christian. Uganda has an agrarian economy with over 80 per cent of the population deriving their livelihood from the agricultural sector. Uganda is recognized by the United Nations as a 'least developed country'. The Uganda National Household Survey 2002/03 indicates that the percentage of people living in poverty stands at 38 per cent, corresponding to 8.9 million Ugandans. This marks a significant increase in poverty both in percentage and absolute terms since 1999/2000. Between 1999/2000 and 2002/03, the incidence of poverty increased more in rural areas than in urban areas (Republic of Uganda, 2006: 22).

Since 2000 there has been significant research undertaken into violence against women in sub-Saharan Africa (Koenig *et al.*, 2003). Using data collected as part of a collaborative intervention to understand and reduce transmission of HIV/AIDS in rural Uganda, Koenig and colleagues (2003) explore the issue of domestic violence from a community-based perspective. The study included the experiences of 5,109 sexually active women of reproductive age who lived in 46 communities in the Rakai district, a rural area in southwestern Uganda that borders the United Republic of Tanzania and Lake Victoria. The Rakai district is dominated by agricultural production, engaging most men and women, education levels are low (particularly for women), and marriage patterns are patrilineal, with women marrying into and residing in their husband's clan. Cultural norms (acceptance of multiple sexual partners among men and polygamous unions) and lack of information concerning HIV has placed the district at the centre of the HIV epidemic in Uganda.

The study found high levels of both verbal abuse (40.1 per cent over the lifetime and 31.3 per cent over the past twelve months) and physical violence (24.8 per cent over the lifetime and 15.1 per cent over the past twelve months). Women's experience of violence was often ongoing, with 60 per cent of those who reported violence during the preceding year reporting three or more specific violent acts in this period (Koenig *et al.*, 2003: 55–6). During the twelve months before the survey, 21.5 per cent of women required medical attention for their injuries at least once.

The research found that most socio-demographic variables had 'limited explanatory contribution', with the exception of high levels of female education (which had a protective effect). 'Risk' factors included: consensual unions (not legally married); relationships of shorter duration (less than five years); alcohol consumption; higher HIV risk; and becoming sexually active at a young age (under fifteen years).

Table 9.2 highlights the common 'reasons' given by women for the violence they experienced. In all but one of these 'reasons' women's actions are seen to contribute directly to their experience of violence.

The research found considerable cultural acceptance of violence against women, with age and gender differences. Women in general were more condoning of violence against women, as were younger people. Young people of both sexes tended to hold views that condone violence against women, a disturbing finding for the future success of intervention programmes (see Table 9.3).

The research concludes that 'episodes of violence are neither infrequent nor isolated events' in rural Uganda and 'little progress in reducing levels of domestic violence is likely to be achieved without significant changes in prevailing individual and community attitudes toward domestic violence' (Koenig *et al.*, 2003: 59).

Adopting an ecological framework, the 'outer circles' encompassing the exosystem and the microsystem provide conceptual grip to the experiences of Ugandan women documented in this study. Interestingly, the individual personal history was seen as being of limited explanatory use. Instead the study highlighted the cultural acceptance of violence against women, informed by beliefs about male dominance in relationships, concepts of ownership and threats to the masculine sense of honour. These were all embedded in a widespread acceptance of physical punishment as a means of dealing with conflict. The level of acceptance of wife bashing among women suggests that the immediate context in which abuse takes place (the micro level) may also be violence-supporting. Extended family members, particularly mothers-in-law, confirm this through their involvement and encouragement of violence.

Bangladesh

Bangladesh is one of the most populous countries in the world on a relatively small land mass. Its population combined with its vulnerability to nature disasters has also made it one of the world's poorest countries. Subsistence farming dominates the rural landscape, although the lives of the rural poor in Bangladesh are

Table 9.2   Primary reasons for assault among 1,014 women reporting recent male against female domestic violence, Rakai District, Uganda, 2000–01

Reasons cited for violence	Women reporting violence (%)
Woman neglected household chores	28.8
Woman disobeyed husband/elders	24.3
Woman's refusal of sex	17.4
Arguments over money	13.5
Suspected infidelity by woman	13.4

Source: Koenig *et al.*, 2003: 57–8

being transformed by micro-credit loan schemes, educational opportunities provided by non-government schools and other progressive interventions (Walker and Matin, 2006). Historically Bangladesh culture is traditional, with strong adherence to the Muslim religion, widespread payment of dowries and strict gender roles although gender roles, like other social and economic aspects, are undergoing rapid change. Bates and colleagues argue that: 'In response to economic necessity, new opportunities and changing norms, women are increasingly deviating from traditional roles, developing new aspirations and, often unintentionally, challenging the prevailing gender order' (Bates *et al.*, 2004: 197).

Since the early 1990s studies have consistently highlighted unacceptably high levels of violence against rural women in Bangladesh. In 1992, 42 per cent of rural married women reported having experienced physical violence at the hands of their husband (Koenig *et al.*, 2003). A more recent study undertaken in 2002 of 1,212 married women in six typical villages found a startling 67 per cent of respondents ever having experienced domestic violence and one-third of women reported ever having experienced major violence (involving kicks, burns or use of weapons). Slightly more than one-third had experienced violence in the past year and 17 per cent had experienced at least one episode of major violence in the past year (Bates *et al.*, 2004: 194–5).

This study supported the 'possible determinants' of Bangladesh's women's vulnerability to violence identified in previous research. A number of factors were identified that increased women's vulnerability to violence in the past year, including:

- dowry arrangements – 45 per cent of women with dowry agreements experienced domestic violence compared to 25 per cent who didn't have an agreement
- marriage registration – 39 per cent of women with a registered marriage experienced domestic violence compared to 28 per cent of those who didn't.
- women's education – 36 per cent of women with less than 5 years' education experienced domestic violence compared to 30 per cent of women with more than 5 years' education

Table 9.3　Attitudes of men and women towards domestic violence, Rakai District, Uganda, 2000–01

Reason	Men	Women
Refusing sex	16	28
Using contraception	22	27
Neglecting household	37	37
Disobeying family	42	50
Infidelity	60	87
Any of the above	70	90

Source: Koenig *et al.*, 2003: 57–8

- women's contribution to covering household expenses – 42 per cent of women who covered household expenses with their own income experienced domestic violence compared to 33 per cent who didn't.

(Bates *et al.*, 2004: 195)

Bates and colleagues argue the centrality of the institution of marriage to rural women's experience of violence: 'marriage related norms and practices reinforce women's relative powerlessness, often exposing them to domestic violence' (Bates *et al.*, 2004: 190–1). The median age at marriage for rural women (aged 20–49) was 15 years in a 1999–2000 national survey (Bates *et al.*, 2004: 191). Young women are often married in childhood to an older man who is unknown to them. Domestic violence is often used by men to establish their dominance and enforce non-egalitarian gender roles early in marriage. These marriage practices are symbolic of male 'ownership' of women. From an ecological perspective, these marriage practices reflect rigid gender expectations enforced through masculine dominance and violence, embedded in the fourth ring or macrosystem. Despite condemning the practice, women interviewed for the study believed the payment of a dowry provided young women with social legitimacy and security. It was recognized as a tool of resource extraction and exploitation but reluctantly perpetuated:

If a girl brings dowry, then she has a stronger position in her in-laws' home … Her mother-in-law cannot torture her, nor can her husband beat her. If they do she can say, 'Did I come here empty-handed?'

(Bates *et al.*, 2004: 193)

Initiatives to empower rural women such as increased education, micro-credit lending, employment initiatives and marriage registration have had perverse effects, with men responding with violence to a woman's increased power and assertiveness. Women's independence, through income or employment, destabilize existing gender norms embedded in the fourth ring or macrosystem. The rather sobering conclusion reached by the study was that:

Changes that somewhat empower women may lead to violence in the near term. Such changes may become protective only after a critical threshold of empowerment has been reached and gender roles have shifted substantially.

(Bates *et al.*, 2004: 197)

Implications for human service providers

The ecological framework provides explanatory insight into the factors that shape rural women's experience of violence. It also provides pointers to the types of interventions that might most usefully prevent violence against rural women in the longer term. The three countries profiled in this chapter – Australia, Uganda and Bangladesh – reveal the complexity of the task. The exo- and macrosystems contribute to enabling and denying violence against rural women in all three countries. In addition to paying attention to the individuals (first layer) and families (second layer), human service providers need to focus on reforming the exo- and macrosystems. The explicit support of violence against women found in the Ugandan study highlights the importance of strengthening informal support systems that reject male violence and support women experiencing violence. If violence against women is seen as acceptable within broader social systems and accepted as a cultural norm, individual women will find it extremely difficult to escape. The poor responses from formal systems such as police and health workers found in the Australian context highlights the need to work at changing organizational cultures that implicitly condone violence against women.

In conclusion, rural women experiencing violence have many of the same issues affecting women living in other settings. The strong community ties, isolation/distance and poor service response, however, created unique difficulties for these women in escaping violence.

Chapter summary

Violence against women in rural settings

- There is a need for caution when using concepts such as 'rural' and 'community'.
- The dominant construction of 'rural communities' renders invisible the divisions of power, privilege, disempowerment and deprivation present within all communities.
- The conceptual 'grip' is provided by an ecological framework in understanding violence against rural women.
- The experiences of women in three very different countries – Australia, Uganda and Bangladesh – reveal that women's experience is strongly influenced by what could be conceived as the 'outer rings' of an ecological framework: the exosystem and macrosystem factors.
- The challenge facing human service providers is needing to be attentive to all four embedded circles concurrently if violence against women in rural settings is to be prevented.

Part III
Violence, abuse and oppression – across the spectrum

10 Violence against children within the family

Fran Waugh

The World Health Organization's (WHO) latest reports on *Violence Against Children* (Pinheiro, 2006) and *Preventing Child Maltreatment: A Guide to Action and Generating Evidence* (WHO and International Society for Child Abuse and Neglect [ISPCAN], 2006) together with UNICEF's (2006) report on *The State of the World's Children, 2007*, emphasize a worldwide obligation to address violence (including domestic violence), abuse and oppression against children as a matter of urgency. Worldwide, children experience a range of violence. For instance: up to 275 million children are estimated to witness domestic violence annually (UNICEF, 2006: 24); in 2002, 150 million girls and 73 million boys under 18 experienced forced sexual intercourse or other forms of sexual violence (Pinheiro, 2006: 14). Studies from many countries in all regions of the world suggest that over 80 per cent of children experience physical punishment in their homes, with at least a third suffering severe physical punishment (Pinheiro, 2006: 14); and in 2002 almost 53,000 children died as a result of homicide (Pinheiro, 2006: 14).

Violence against children is prevalent and increasing in all countries. It has a devastating impact upon children's health, welfare, emotional wellbeing, life chances and safety. This knowledge is not new to democratic capitalist countries as evidenced over the past forty years by a plethora of agencies, policy and practice strategies, reports, research, training and community education, in attempting to understand and be responsive to this social problem. However, this is a highly sensitive and political issue, where non-accidental deaths of children are to be prevented at all costs. Parents' and governments' responsibilities for children's rights to provision, protection and participation outlined in the United Nations Convention on the Rights of the Child, 1989 (Alderson, 2003) are compromised by limited resources. In addition, incorporating lessons learnt from recent research and practice about the complex, multidimensional nature of violence, abuse and oppression against children and how this can be addressed, remains a challenge.

This chapter focuses on violence against children within the family in democratic capitalist countries, in particular Australia, the United Kingdom (UK) and the United States of America (USA). The family continues to be a main site for abuse and neglect of children (Dowd, 2006). Key concepts related to risk, protection and resilience often feature in practice, policy and research discussions about violence against children in the family home (Fraser, Richman and Galinsky, 1999; Gillingham, 2006), the subject of this chapter. Debates related to risk, protection and resilience, focus on definitional issues, rights and responsibilities. Challenges include developing policies and practices which are evidence-based and are cognizant of the complexities of children's and parents' lives; poverty and social disadvantage; gender issues; the need for meaningful participation of children and parents and the development of effectual partnerships between key players, including children, parents, practitioners, policy makers, researchers, educators and politicians. Initially, a snapshot is provided of the level of violence against children in the family to demonstrate that such violence continues to be a major social concern. This is followed by an outline of the underlying discourses, namely, human rights, public health, ecological and feminists' perspectives which provide the parameters for the discussion in this chapter.

A snapshot: the level of violence against children in families

This chapter follows the United Nations Convention on the Rights of the Child and defines a child as encompassing the period from birth to 18 years of age. Debates as to how countries or even states within countries define violence against children are ongoing. Poverty is a major factor contributing to the oppression of children (UNICEF, 2006) which is addressed in Chapter 4, 'Trapped within poverty and violence'. This chapter adopts a definition of violence against children which is comprehensive, including physical abuse, sexual abuse, psychological abuse, neglect and/or domestic violence. Children are oppressed by such experiences because of misuse of power by a trusted person, usually the father or father figure in experiences of sexual abuse, domestic violence, psychological abuse, serious physical abuse and child homicides (Corby, 2000; Calder, Harold and Howarth, 2004; Cavanagh, Dobash and Dobash, 2005; Radford and Hester, 2006). For this reason the main emphasis of this chapter is on men who perpetrate abuse against their children and women rather than mothers or siblings who perpetrate abuse. This, however, does not detract from the importance of men being responsible fathers which is addressed in Chapter 3, 'Men and violence'.

The number of children as victims of abuse and neglect in the family home is increasing (Waldfogel, 1998; Liddell, Donegan, Goddard and Tucci, 2006; Scott, 2006; Australian Institute of Health and Welfare [AIHW], 2007). An examination of the number of official reports of child abuse and neglect in the United States and Australia paint a picture of an escalating number of reports. In the United States in 1967 there were less than 10,000 reports of child abuse and neglect, rising to more than 1.8 million reports in 2002 (Waldfogel, 1998: 104; Pecora, Whittaker and Maluccio, 2006). There were 1,400 children who died as a result of abuse or neglect in the United States in 2002 (Pecora Whittaker *et al.*, 2006). As Scott (2006) notes international comparative policy analysis in child protection is difficult because of significant difference in child abuse data and broader social and economic contexts. However, in the 1990s the United States had three times the rate of reports, four times the rate of child abuse deaths and twice the rate of children in state care as the United Kingdom. In England and Wales there are estimated to be 376,000 children in need, defined as 'children whose development is impaired or likely to be impaired or who are disabled and in need of services' (Rose, Gray and McAuley 2006, p.21).

In Australia reports to the child protection system more than doubled from 107,134 in 1999–2000 to 266,745 in 2005–6 (AIHW, 2007). Indigenous children are over-represented in child protection systems in Australia, being five times more likely to be the subject of substantiation than other children, six times more likely to be placed on care and protection orders and seven times more likely to be placed in out-of-home care (AIHW, 2007). In 2002 it was estimated in the United States that 17 million children (out of a possible 72.9 million) lived in families with incomes below the poverty line compared with 3.66 million children (out of a possible 11.9 million) in the United Kingdom in 2003. Increasing public awareness about child abuse, neglect and domestic violence, mandatory reporting by professionals in Australia and the United States and the widening of reportable categories, for instance including domestic violence as a child 'at risk' matter, provide partial explanation for the escalating number of reports.

Ways of understanding child abuse, neglect and domestic violence

There are multiple ideologies, values and beliefs operating in child protection and child welfare agencies about children and families and multiple theoretical perspectives which inform understandings about child abuse, neglect and domestic violence. Domestic violence is discussed in detail in the Chapter 2, 'Women and violence', and in all the chapters in Part II. Therefore, while this discussion focuses on child abuse and neglect, it does not exclude the importance of understanding the links between child abuse and neglect and domestic violence.

Corby notes child abuse and neglect is dependent upon the cultural context and the dominant discourse which informs our understandings (Corby, 2000: 66). For instance, legal, human rights, public health, child protection, psychological (individual and interactionist), sociological (socio-cultural, socio-structural and feminist) discourses may underpin definitions and understandings about child abuse and neglect (Corby, 2000: 132–55). The theoretical basis of policy and practice in child abuse and neglect shifted from a dominant medical discourse of individual pathology in the 1960s through to the interactive, sociological, socio-cultural and ecological perspectives in the 1970s and 1980s, and to feminists, human rights, consumer rights, needs and risk discourse and public health in the late 1980s, 1990s and early 2000s (Belsky, 1978; Harrold, 1987; Pardeck, 1989; MacKinnon, 1992; Humphreys, 1993; O'Hagan and Dillenburger, 1995; Waugh, 1997; Waterson, 1999; Corby, 2000; D'Cruz, 2004; Millar and Corby, 2006; Scott, 2006; WHO and ISPCAN, 2006).

As mentioned previously this chapter is influenced by human rights, public health, ecological and feminist perspectives which view the abuse and neglect of children as the result of human actions, beliefs, behaviours and circumstances which have been formed and influenced by a range of factors including the conditions under which adults and children live, cultural beliefs about children, gender, ethnicity, the influence of power, economic circumstances (poverty), the adult's own parenting experiences, personality and family relations (Garbarino, 1981; Munro, 2005; WHO and ISPCAN, 2006). These perspectives inform how dimensions of risk, protection and resilience are understood.

For instance the human rights perspective encompasses the rights of all children to safety, welfare and wellbeing. Within such a human rights perspective, governments in partnership with non-government agencies and the community at large, aim to ensure the safety, welfare and wellbeing of children through the provision of a range of economic, social, health, child protection, welfare services and resources. The ultimate goal is the creation of a just society which promotes and enhances the development of children to their maximum potential. This means the absence of child abuse, neglect and domestic violence and reducing risk factors which cumulatively contribute to violence against children and the enhancement of protective factors.

The ecological perspective views individual differences, family influences, community influences and cultural influences as interacting with and contributing to, the aetiology of child abuse and neglect (Garbarino, 1981; Iverson and Segal, 1990; Cooper, 1993; WHO and ISPCAN, 2006). Therefore, in relation to risk, it is important not only to identify the different areas but also how they are interacting and resulting in cumulative risk. Likewise, to increase protection for children, the different areas and their interaction need to be understood.

The public health perspective, based on the health promotion ideals of strengths and assets, aims to increase community capacity to address child abuse and neglect through the use of existing social capital in universal services such as early childhood programmes (Scott 2006). In this perspective action is taken to: prevent violence against children from occurring; detect cases and intervene early; provide ongoing care to victims and families where violence occurs; and prevent the reoccurrence of violence (WHO and ISPCAN, 2006). It acknowledges the importance of applying a holistic, multi-pronged approach which includes prevention, community education, community development, early intervention, statutory and non-statutory intervention, and follow-up assistance regarding child abuse and neglect (Scott, 2006). By adopting such a multi-pronged approach risk factors can be identified and addressed, and protection factors can be increased to lessen the chance of violence against children. This approach is dependent upon agreement about risk factors between the multiple players. This is an area of possible contention which will be considered in the later discussion.

Feminist perspectives highlight the significance of gender, power and race in abusive relationships (Corby, 2000; Daniel, Featherstone, Hooper and Scourfield, 2005; Humphreys and Stanley, 2006; Radford and Hester, 2006; UNICEF, 2006).

These elements are critical in understanding the dynamics of risk and protection. For instance, studies from Canada, the United States, the United Kingdom and Australia indicate a strong correlation between violence against women and violence against children (UNICEF, 2006). Such knowledge about the co-existence of domestic violence and child abuse and neglect and the effects that domestic violence has on mothering (Edleson, 1999; Mullender, Hague, Imam, *et al.*, 2002; Calder *et al.*, 2004; Humphreys and Stanley, 2006; Radford and Hester, 2006), is vital in addressing violence against children in a holistic manner. It is imperative that such knowledge underpins concepts of risk, protection and resilience which are operating in prevention, intervention and recovery strategies.

Risk, protection and resilience: definitional issues, rights and responsibilities

The language of risk stretches over a range of social activities, practices and experiences with its material consequences remaining contestable (Mythen and Walklate, 2006: 1). According to Beck the concept of risk 'characterizes a peculiar, intermediate state between security and destruction, where the *perception* of threatening risks determines thought and action' (2000: 213). In the area of child abuse, neglect and domestic violence, 'risk' together with 'protection' have become salient concepts for understanding and responding to experiences of victims of violence and perpetrators of violence. How risk, protection and resilience are defined has important implications for policies and practices in shaping prevention, intervention and recovery strategies with children and their families. Definitions of risks have been linked with concepts of harm or danger or as a chance to gain benefits in a situation where harm is also possible (Alaszewski, 1998). Such terms as reduction, containment, minimization and prediction feature in discussion about risk. The meanings attributed to risk may differ between the various players in the child protection context, for instance practitioners and parents may have different perceptions about risk. For example in a situation where children are living with domestic violence the risks perceived by the children, parents, statutory and non-statutory practitioners may vary (Irwin, Waugh and Wilkinson, 2000; Houghton, 2006; Mullender, 2006). Definitions can be operationalized along a continuum from a narrow focus at one end to a broader focus at the other end (Waugh 2006).

In narrow definitions the emphasis is placed on individual events, for example a physical abuse incident, a sexual abuse incident or an incident of domestic violence. In these situations risk is equated to harm and the negative outcomes of the event. The context of the event and the relevant history is not elicited or the likelihood of future harm is not considered. Whereas in the broader definitions, a more comprehensive assessment, based on ecological and feminist perspectives, is undertaken. For example, this comprises taking into account factors related to the child (age, gender, development functioning, behaviour, their presentation, their understanding of the incident causing the harm), the parents (attitudes to harm and to their child, relationship to the child and other family members, functioning, parenting capacity, disability, presence of domestic violence, level of power, responsibilities and blame), the environment (whether basic needs in terms of housing, food, clothing, education, medical needs are being met), the community (formal and informal networks in the community) and cultural factors (Gillingham, 2006; Waugh, 2006). For instance risk is associated with adolescent parents; lesser levels of education; learning difficulties; living in unstable, transient relationships; and a history of inadequate care and abuse, mental health issues, disability issues, drug and alcohol misuse (Bentovim, 2006). Environmental risk factors may include living in poverty, overcrowding, substandard housing, unemployment, isolation in the community from wider family, and poorly resourced communities (Bentovim, 2006).

The purposes of risk assessments in child protection have been challenged and are not always viewed as resulting in a positive outcome for the child and their family (Gillingham, 2006). There is debate as to whether child protection statutory authorities should adopt actuarial, consensus or professional judgement models of risk assessment. While all three models are claimed to be evidence-based, actuarial models are often criticized for being mechanistic and prescriptive as workers add up scores to determine the overall level of risk. Minimal value is placed on the importance of professional judgement and the analytical skills of workers to make sense of complex situations (Waugh, 2006). In professional judgement models, based on the practitioner's analysis of the severity of the incident, the vulnerability of the child, the likelihood of it happening again (in light of for example: the family history, domestic violence, mental health or drug and alcohol misuse) and as well as safety aspects, practitioners are required to make a professional judgement about existing harm and its consequences and the probability of future harm (Dalgleish, 2004). A statement about immediate safety and possible consequences of intervention is required. The focus is on balancing negative consequences against positive outcomes and guarding against the likelihood of harm in the future (Dalgleish, 2004).

In order to get away from the narrow focus of risk assessment the government in England and Wales developed an assessment framework based on three systems, namely the child's developmental needs (such as, health, educational, emotional, family and social relationships) the parents' capacities to respond appropriately to those needs (such as providing basic care, ensuring safety, emotional warmth, stability) and family history, wider family and environmental factors (such as housing, employment, income, family's social integration and community resources) (Rose, 2006). However, if there are excessive unmet needs, these could be framed as risks or if they are addressed then these could be viewed as protective aspects. This is not to suggest that there is a linear relationship between needs, risks and protection.

Beck posits that 'risks only suggest what should *not* be done, not what *should* be done' (2000: 218). It is argued that protective factors and processes, while conceptually distinctive from risk factors, modify risk and suggest what should be done (Rutter 1987 in Fraser *et al.*, 1999). Like risk factors, protective factors may be found in individual characteristics (for example, an easy-going temperament, tenacity, responsibility, insight, independence, initiative, creativity, humour), family factors (for example, empathy, parental warmth and supervision) or extra-familial conditions (for example, having a network of supportive friends) (Rutter, 1987; Fraser *et al.*, 1999). Factors that are likely to be protective in the home include good parenting, the development of strong attachment bonds between parents and children and positive non-violent discipline (Pinheiro, 2006).

Resilience, in contrast, denotes positive adaptation and competence despite the presence of substantial risk (Fraser *et al.*, 1999). It is defined by Grotberg as 'A universal capacity which allows a person, group or community to prevent, mini-mize or overcome the damaging effects of adversity' (1997: 19, cited in Hester, Pearson and Harwin, 2007: 83). Three aspects of resilience purported by Fraser and colleagues (1999) are: overcoming the odds (children who thrive despite exposure to high risk such as living with domestic violence), maintaining compe-tence when faced with pressure (such as ongoing domestic violence) and recov-ering from trauma (overcoming negative life experiences such as physical abuse, sexual abuse and emotional abuse through informal and formal assistance). In each of these aspects, resilience is characterized by successful functioning in the context of high risk.

Resilience factors have also been described by some authors as adaptive processes internal to the child while protective factors and processes exist in the environment (Smokowski, 1998). Other researchers claim that protective mecha-nisms promote resilience by interacting with risk factors. In other words, protec-tive processes comprises the factors in the child's environment that act as a buffer to the negative effects of adverse experiences (Daniel, Wassell and Gilligan, 1999). Bentovim in his discussion on therapeutic interventions with children who have experienced sexual and physical abuse, notes that,

> Children are more resilient if they have higher levels of intelligence, health and attractiveness, or if they have a supportive parent, sibling or extended family member or adequate support in the community with well-developed universal and targeted services.
>
> (Bentovim, 2006: 145)

Cree and Wallace (2005) discuss rights, responsibilities and values in relation to risk and protection. They argue that while risk and protection are 'perceived differently by different people at different times risk can have serious conse-quences for children and their families' (Cree and Wallace, 2005: 127). For instance, in assessing the rights and responsibilities in a domestic violence sit-uation, such a position takes away the double blame mothers often experience because of 'gender entrapment'. Radford and Hester (2006) point out that mothers are frequently blamed for the risks their children experience by being exposed to domestic violence and for not protecting their children from the influence of the perpetrator of violence. As Humphreys and Stanley (2006), Mullender (2006), and Radford and Hester (2006) highlight, intervention needs to focus on the perpetrator and ensure that the mother is fully supported in ways which help her.

Parents are held to be responsible for providing 'good enough' care for their children and to minimize harmful risks in their children's lives. In terms of the responsibilities of governments to address risk, there are multiple strategies ranging from universal resources to address poverty, to prevention, early intervention and community development programmes which target children and their families where risks have been identified prior to any incidents of child abuse and neglect taking place. There are also specialized child protection services to investigate allegations of child abuse and neglect and specialized treatment/recovery services and legal services to assist children to deal with abuse and neglect and to prevent re-abuse.

The challenges: risk, protection and resilience

It is important to consider the context in which interests in risks, protective factors and resilience regarding violence against children in the family home, has flourished.

There has been an underlying shift from purely child protection orientation (such as in the USA and Canada) focusing on protecting children from abusive parents to child welfare or family services orientation (found in Germany and Finland) aimed at understanding situations and acts which are considered harmful to children in the context of the difficulties experienced by families, such as living in poverty (Spratt, 2001). In addition there are countries which encompass aspects of both (such as the United Kingdom and Australia) (Spratt, 2001). This means broadening the net of intervention from merely focusing on an incident of abuse and assigning individual blame and responsibility (investigation focus) to adopting a more comprehensive response and offering prevention and early intervention and recovery strategies to address identified issues.

Ideally, strategies to achieve optimal intervention and outcomes for children and their families are informed by relevant evidence, based on sound quantitative and qualitative research and practice wisdom (Macdonald, 2001). Such evidence has focused on ways of understanding: the children's experience of abuse, neglect and/or domestic violence; mothers' experiences; fathers' experiences (predominately the perpetrator of abuse); sibling's experiences; community attitudes about children, parenting and discipline; and the impact of various interventions. Such research has increased knowledge and understanding about ways of minimizing risk and increasing protective processes. For instance in the United Kingdom there have been literature reviews of research on child protection, child deaths (Cavanagh *et al.*, 2005), residential care, supporting parents, the effectiveness of child welfare interventions and community based initiatives, child protection outcomes and the costs of child welfare intervention (Pecora, McAuley and Rose, 2006). In the United States and Canada reviews have focused on evidence on the effectiveness of child welfare interventions, on early childhood interventions, home visiting services, family support, child maltreatment including the impact of physical punishment (Gershoff, 2002), the impact of domestic violence (Edleson, 1999), multisystemic family theory, family foster care and residential care (Pecora, McAuley *et al.*, 2006). In Australia there has been a national audit of child protection and out-of-home care research (Cashmore, Higgins, Bromfield and Scott, 2006). This audit highlights many unanswered questions about the dynamics of parent, child and family behaviours and how best to address those that may be harmful (Tomison, 2002; Cashmore, *et al.*, 2006; Liddell *et al.*, 2006).

What has become evident through the vast literature on child abuse, neglect and/or domestic violence over the past forty years is the complexity of the lives of children and their families, the multidimensional and dynamic nature of the abuse and neglect which children experience, the gendered nature of the abuse and domestic violence, and the diversity and ongoing uncertainty which characterizes the lives of these children (Pinheiro, 2006). Such complexity may involve families where child abuse, neglect and/or domestic violence is intersected with one or a combination of the following dimensions: parents living with a mental illness which negatively impacts on their parenting ability (Stanley, Penhale, Riordan, Barbour and Holden, 2003; Humphreys and Stanley, 2006), parental drug and/or alcohol misuse (Humphreys, Regan, River and Thiara, 2005; Hegarty, 2004;), disability issues, lack of financial resources due to unemployment and limited educational opportunities, lack of adequate housing, diminished social networks (Humphreys and Stanley, 2006; Scott, 2006; WHO and ISPCAN, 2006); and communities with multiple disadvantage which are under-resourced (Garbarino, 1992; Vinson, 2007). These problems are compounded for Indigenous children where families and communities experienced legacies of oppressive colonial policies and practices (for example, Indigenous children in Australia and Canada, and children in South Africa whose parents experienced the apartheid policies) (HREOC, 1997; Bird, 1998; Gordon, Hallahan and Henry, 2002; September, 2006). See Chapter 5, 'Towards healing: recognizing the trauma surrounding Aboriginal family violence, for more detail.

Despite increases in funding to child welfare services tensions remain in Australia about the chronic under-resourcing of child abuse, neglect and domestic violence services (Liddell *et al.*, 2006). This is often coupled with practitioners experiencing difficult conditions of practice in terms of lack of organizational support (Conrad and Kellar-Guenther, 2006; De Panfallis, 2006). In addition workers are required to manage the stress associated with intervening in the most difficult and complex situations in the lives of children where violence is occurring in the family (Stanley and Goddard, 2002). See also Chapter 16, 'Human service professionals: violence and the workplace'.

Implications for human service professionals

Children who experience abuse, neglect and/or domestic violence and their families require a range of tailored, multi-level interventions ascertained through comprehensive needs and risk assessments based on the skills, values, knowledge and understanding of professionals within a legislative framework (Waterson, 1999; Cree and Wallace, 2005; Millar and Corby, 2006). Until recently discussions on risk and protection in Australia and the United States have focused predominately on statutory child protection interventions. However, within human rights, ecological, public health and feminist perspectives, a much wider net has been cast to include prevention, early intervention and recovery strategies. This has also provided the basis for broadening researchers', policy makers' and practitioners' understandings about resilience-based practice models which mobilize key protective processes that buffer the child or family against risk (Smokowski, 1998: 337).

It is important therefore for practitioners, policy makers, educators and researchers to be aware of where they would place themselves along the continuum of narrow versus broad definitions of risk. How do their own values and personal experiences influence their understandings about risk and harm and in particular what do they include as risk factors? It is equally important for the different players to be aware of how the parameters of risk are shaped by the agency and by the legislation which underpins their practice (Cree and Wallace, 2005; Waugh, 2006). For instance, child protection practitioners, health practitioners, police officers and legal practitioners need to be able to critically unpack these areas and to consider how these interact with their own operational definitions. In addition, throughout intervention with children and families, practitioners need to understand that the child and the family might interpret risk differently. Due to the changing evidence available, for instance through research and practice wisdom, the different players do not necessarily have a fixed, static position about risk but rather their positions may change depending on the particular context. This notion of fluid definitions then further complicates the already complex situations faced by practitioners when working with children and families where child protection issues are raised. Throughout this dynamic process of defining risk, the rights of the child, need to be clearly emphasized.

Because of the complex and diverse family contexts of child abuse, neglect and/or domestic violence, a wide range of interventions are required. Research has highlighted the importance of adopting a multi-sectoral approach where coordination and collaboration are key in providing optimal intervention when responding to child abuse, neglect and/or domestic violence (van Eyk and Baum, 2002; NSW Government 2006; Richardson and Asthana, 2006). For instance a 'whole of government approach' to children and families has been adopted in New South Wales (NSW), Australia and the United Kingdom have adopted an 'integrated' and 'joined-up' approach to working with children and families (NSW Government, 2006; Rose *et al.*, 2006).

Partnerships between workers from different agencies and appropriate participation by children and their families have also been identified as key ingredients in ensuring positive interventions where risks are minimized and protective factors increased (Tucci, Mitchell and Goddard, 2006; Stanley *et al.*, 2003; Hegarty, 2004; NSW Government, 2006; Humphreys and Stanley, 2006; Radford and Hester, 2006;). In addition to coordination and collaboration, time and time again research has highlighted the need for workers in different agencies to have open communication with each other and with the child and their family to ensure the most appropriate decisions are made. Some instances where this has not happened have been documented in reports on reviewable child deaths (Munro, 2005; NSW Ombudsman, 2006).

Practitioners need to ensure that they: find ways of talking to children; make time to listen to children and to build relationships with them, avoid imposing their views on the child but elicit the child's understanding of a situation and what they see their protection needs as being (Mullender *et al.*, 2002; Calder *et al.*, 2004; Aubrey and Dahl, 2006; Connolly, Crichton-Hill and ward, 2006; Houghton, 2006). Also the involvement of the child's family members as active participants addressing responsibility and power issues is considered vital to the success of any intervention programme (Radford and Hester, 2006; Rose *et al.*, 2006). Campbell (1997: 8) notes that in the process of assessing child-at-risk concerns active participation by family members requires professionals to demonstrate their willingness to inform and listen respectfully, to give full and frank information of their assessment, to hear the family's views and to look with them at the resources they have at their disposal, what they feel they need and how these can be appropriately linked with available services and resources.

National standards for intervention with children and families have been developed in England and Wales resulting in 'joined-up' working between services where common assessment frameworks underpin intervention services to ensure sharper, more open and transparent decision-making with clear lines of accountability (Rose *et al.*, 2006). The emphasis is on identifying and responding to needs and enhancing protection, thereby reducing risk. It would be useful to consider the applicability of developing national standards in the Australian context of state-based child protection legislation. Furthermore, ways of nurturing meaningful participation of children and parents to promote partnerships between them and service providers is important (Houghton, 2006) in facilitating how risk is minimized and managed, protection enhanced and resilience fostered.

The extent to which policy makers and practitioners can remain up-to-date with the ever-increasing evidence, is variable. This is dependent upon the value the worker places on ongoing life-long learning, and how they make sense of the new material and understand the implications of it for their practice. Just as critical is a work culture which values and facilitates evidence-based practice by providing time to workers to access material, attend training and conferences and participate in research. For instance the New South Wales, Department of Community Services (statutory child protection authority) established a Practice Research unit as a means of disseminating information to their current child and family workers in early intervention, intake (helpline), investigation, follow-up and out-of-home care. The challenge is for workers to achieve a balance between the continual demands of their day-to-day practice and their responsibility to incorporate current relevant research in their practice. In this way they can ensure that they are not only able to identify risks and needs but to respond in ways that enhance the protection and safety of children and their families.

In conclusion, theory, policy and practice in relation to addressing violence, abuse and oppression against children in the family has seen a number of important developments in our understandings about the complexity and diversity of the multiple interacting factors contributing to the causes of this violence. Violence against children in the family remains a complex issue for governments to address worldwide. Addressing poverty and alienation in communities which experience multiple disadvantage remain a major challenge. Another challenge is to cross-fertilize knowledge and understanding about the way children experience violence in other contexts such as in schools, in countries experiencing conflict and war, in places of employment, in people trafficking and in the sex industry.

In Australia, the United Kingdom and the United States, multiple strategies have been developed and implemented either explicitly or implicitly to minimize risk, increase protection and nurture resilience in response to violence against children in the family. Micro and macro dimensions of risk have been identified where child abuse and neglect occur, but less is know about the interaction of protection and the enhancement of resilience. Complexities and uncertainties continue to abound in the lives of children and their families where there are concerns of child abuse, neglect and/or domestic violence. This requires policy makers and practitioners to exercise the highest level of professionalism to ensure that the most relevant knowledge and skills inform their practice. Most importantly in our global society it requires sharing of knowledge and analysis of evidence to determine which is applicable between countries given the differences in cultures, histories, values, intervention approaches, policies and programme structures (Pecora, McAuley *et al.*, 2006). It requires that organizations provide supportive structures and processes to facilitate this. It requires researchers to explore and examine the questions raised by policy makers, practitioners, children and their families. Participation and partnership of children and their families is called upon not only at the intervention stage but also at the policy development stage and in setting the research agenda. It is only through listening to children and their families in ways that are meaningful that increased understanding about protection and enhancing resilience can be achieved. This then can be woven into future strategies to address violence against children (Akister, 2006).

Chapter summary

Violence against children within the family

- Violence against children is prevalent and increasing in all countries.
- Violence has a devastating impact upon children's health, welfare, emotional wellbeing, life chances and safety.
- The family continues to be a main site of abuse, neglect and/or domestic violence for children.
- Human rights, public health discourse, risk discourse, ecological and feminists' perspectives underpin strategies which address violence against children.
- Key concepts related to risk, protection and resilience often feature in practice, policy and research discussions about violence against children in the family.

(Continued)

- Debates related to risk, protection and resilience, focus on: definitional issues; rights; and responsibilities.
- Challenges related to risk, protection and resilience include developing policies and practices which are evidence-based and are cognizant of: the complexities of children's and parents' lives; poverty and social disadvantage; gender issues; race issues; the need for meaningful participation of children and parents; and the development of effectual partnerships between key players.
- Ways of nurturing meaningful participation of children and parents to promote partnerships between them and service providers is important in facilitating how risk is minimized and managed, protection enhanced and resilience fostered.
- Complexities and uncertainties continue to abound in the lives of children and their families where there are concerns of child abuse, neglect and/or domestic violence. This requires policy makers and practitioners to exercise the highest level of professionalism to ensure that the most relevant knowledge and skills inform their practice.

11 Violence and the state: asylum seeker children

Denise Lynch

> Everyone has the right to seek and to enjoy in other countries asylum from persecution.
>
> (Article 14, Universal Declaration of Human Rights, 1948)

This chapter will address structural violence towards asylum seeker children and consider contributory factors from both an Australian and international perspective. In this chapter it is argued that structural violence is being perpetrated against asylum seeker children following arrival in their country of destination. The evidence for this is shown in their health difficulties, their problems in education, problems in housing and difficulties in income provision. But this structural violence and oppression, caused in some part by their unresolved legal status, has other significant consequences; children cannot develop and form an identity or a sense of belonging with their new country. In the Australian context collateral damage to children, stemming from deliberate state policies and practices focusing on deterrence has meant that, for example, perceptions of Australia as a fair country, where children and families are given a 'fair go' is questionable.

This chapter begins by examining the structural violence and oppression that is perpetrated on children who have come to Australia in the last ten years attempting to gain 'refugee' status. These children are legally regarded as 'asylum seekers', and they have experienced various forms of torture and trauma in their country of origin and in their journey to their 'host' country (Brennan, 2003). Current Australian laws and social policies, combined with a political agenda of deterrence, often means children and families find themselves in great difficulty. They are not able to fully settle in their new country and unable to return to their country of origin while they wait for their legal situation to be resolved. For asylum seeker children these legal difficulties often contribute to problems in education, health (particularly mental health) and most importantly these children are hindered in the development of a sense of identity and belonging with their new country. These difficulties also delay an ability to progress in their new life with security and stability. It is argued that this combination of difficulties constitutes 'structural violence' and it is being perpetrated by the state and mostly sanctioned within the community.

This chapter will concentrate on two major contexts to examine the effects on children and families. These are: asylum seeking children in the community, and asylum seeking children in detention. While it is acknowledged that unaccompanied children have particular needs, the focus of the chapter is with children and their families. This in no way underestimates the difficulties of unaccompanied children (see Kohli, 2006; Thomas, Thomas, Nafees and Bhugra, 2004; McKelvey and Webb,1995). Australia has uniquely detained asylum seekers, including children, and while this practice essentially finished in respect of children in 2005, it still exists for adults, and the ramifications for families and children are therefore still significant. It is also argued that the symbolic significance of this policy goes far beyond the physical implementation.

The chapter has two objectives: one is to indicate the breadth and depth of the structural violence being imposed on children, including identity issues and the other is to understand the root causes of this violence beyond the policy of deterrence. Policies do not operate in isolation and thus the values and philosophy underpinning these policies, needs to be carefully understood so that a range of strategies to reduce harm to children can be considered.

A further major concern linked to both objectives is a largely passive community response to this structural violence against families and children. In fact this response assists with the maintenance of this type of violence, and it could be argued, is relied upon to perpetrate the violence. Judith Herman's work has relevance here. She states

> It is very tempting to take the side of the perpetrator. All the perpetrator asks is that the bystander do nothing. ... In order to escape accountability for his crimes, the perpetrator does everything in his power to promote forgetting. Secrecy and silence are the perpetrator's first line of defense.
>
> (Herman, 1992: 7)

It is also argued that this passive community response is a powerful tool for those in positions of authority making decisions regarding citizenship in Australia.

The evidence of structural violence

Structural violence is defined as:

> forms of institutionalized social injustice, it is an attempt to move beyond the commonsense understanding of violence as the individual use of bodily force. It calls attention to the violence that inheres in some social roles, norms and patterns, as well as to the persistence and durability of those patterns.
>
> (Calhoun, 2002: 590)

Kent (2000) extends this definition as it applies to children:

> Structural violence is harm imposed by some people on others indirectly, through the social system as they pursue their own preferences. It produces

a variety of harms to children, including the massive mortality of children throughout the world.

(Kent, 2000: 2)

Asylum seeker children would appear to many Australians to be unbelievably lucky. Often these children have witnessed death or torture of relatives in their country of origin from which they have escaped and are alive in a western country. They are in a war-free environment, and they have a chance for a 'better life'. Mostly they are with their immediate families. It is almost beyond belief that their life is not good. But there is a growing body of evidence, nationally and internationally (see Fazel and Stein, 2002; Rousseau and Drapeau, 2003; Hodes, 2002), to support the premise that their lives are often extremely difficult.

By saying this, it is not implied that they have arrived in their host country without some major problems. What is being argued is that following arrival, these children and their families experience structural violence as a result of deliberate neglect of their major needs and a complete abrogation of concern for their future. One of the features of Australia's recent refugee policy for persons attempting to gain refugee status has been mandatory detention. Australia has been the only country which has implemented mandatory detention for some arrivals without papers, and until 2005, as highlighted this included children (Mares, 2004). Therefore, children who are 'asylum seekers' in Australia, including those who have been in detention, represent a unique group.

An analysis of this situation for children and families leads to an understanding that the major problems that are being experienced are not an unplanned consequence of old or irrelevant laws, but are the result of factors which are deliberately combined to produce a level of difficulty against this group of people in Australia and in other countries.

Although Australia has mandatory detention and other policies of deterrence, it is not alone internationally. There are policies in the United Kingdom, Germany and the United States which present great difficulties to asylum seekers and their families. Sales states:

> Asylum policy in Britain is preoccupied with control, with no national system for the support of refugees. The new social support system for asylum seekers, particularly the voucher system and compulsory dispersal, serve to isolate them from society and promote intense social exclusion.

(Sales, 2002: 456)

Structural violence and oppression are reduced when asylum seekers are assisted positively by early intervention, particularly with regard to health, education, housing and employment. If there is a welcoming community, and partnerships with services are developed, particularly language services, then structural violence is curtailed considerably (Taylor and Stanovic, 2005; Clark, 2006).

History and political frameworks in Australia

In discussing the issues for asylum seeker children, it is imperative to understand some of the complex history of Australian migration. Social and historical contexts give understanding to the current issues and also can assist explanations of past policy and practice. Obviously, the history of Australia is not the same as other western countries, but in describing Australia's migration history, there are themes that emerge that are relevant for, and similar to, other countries.

Australia, with many other countries, including the United Kingdom, is a signatory to the 1951 Convention Relating to the Status of Refugees, and the 1947 and 1989 United Nations Convention on the Rights of the Child (Australian Department of Immigration and Citizenship, 2007).

Australia has a long history of migration. While having Anglo-Celtic origins, the country has had waves of migration since 1788. Following the Second World War, Australia opened its gates to migrants, primarily from Anglo-Celtic regions, but also from Greece, Italy and the former Yugoslavia, to assist with an emerging industrial workforce to move Australia away from its dependency on agriculture and the sheep industry. Although the existing policy, the White Australia Policy, prevailed, there was a far more diverse migrant intake (Lynch, 2006).

In the 1970s there was a move towards 'integration' in migrant policy with a new Labour government that embraced greater openness. With Australia having a physical proximity to Asia, there was a logical move of many refugees to come to Australia in the 1970s. For many Vietnamese, there was a need to escape political terror and/or poverty (APMRN, 1996). By these 'boat people' arriving there was a strong humanitarian push for appropriate settlement. This followed Australia's contested role in the Vietnam War and a community perception that acceptance of Vietnamese refugees was a necessary moral action (Manne and Corlett, 2004: 4).

The above discussion implies a smooth transition for migrants and refugees. For individuals and groups this was not always the case. Migrants, and more particularly refugees, were not accepted quickly. There was intolerance of those who did not speak English and for many, low-paying work was the inevitable outcome for people with little formal education, or those who did not have 'accredited' qualifications. As stated by Tascon:

> Australia … is deeply inscribed with racialised-exclusions and the need to determine who crosses the borders. It is a need that attempts to protect its whiteness. There are ethnic/religious dimensions to this whiteness – including the preservation of Anglo-Celtic and Judeo-Christian traditions.
> (Tascon, 2002: 3)

In the 1980s and 1990s, there was a further evolution and the policies and laws reflected multiculturalism.

> Australian multiculturalism … recognizes, accepts, respects and celebrates
> our cultural diversity. It embraces the heritage of Indigenous Australians,
> early European settlement, our Australian-grown customs and those of the
> diverse range of migrants now coming to this country.
>
> (Australian Department of Immigration and Multicultural and
> Indigenous Affairs, 2004: 1)

But always there was another parallel reality for people who were perceived as
different or threatening. In the mid-1990s there was the emergence of an independent politician, who spoke openly and negatively about migrants and difference in Australia. Although her term in politics was quite short, she had a great
deal of community support for those views.

In the last ten years, there have been ongoing changes that have affected migration laws and policy and have had serious consequences for asylum seekers and
refugees. The contributing factors to these changes have been global terrorism,
bringing with it a climate of fear, particularly related to the Middle East and radical Islam, and a conservative government, which has developed policies and
laws which limit the rights and freedoms of asylum seekers and refugees.

The consequences of these factors have resulted in a tightening of policies, practices and laws about people trying to enter Australia other than by orthodox means.
This has generally been accepted by the Australian community. Notwithstanding,
there have been a number of writers and community groups that have formally
and informally advocated on behalf of asylum seekers and refugees (for example,
Father Frank Brennan, Robert Manne, the NSW Refugee Council, STARTT,
NSW Asylum Seekers Centre, ChilOut and GetUp). Thus, while community
acceptance has occurred there certainly has been a contested dialogue in the
media between a range of interest groups about what Australia's response to asylum seekers and refugees should be.

Ways of understanding structural violence and oppression

Reference to one single perspective will not assist in the understanding of child
refugees and their experiences of structural violence and oppression. However,
there are a number of conceptual frameworks that combine to give a clearer perspective on the plight of refugee children around the world. Notwithstanding, it
is acknowledged that the orientations discussed in this chapter are 'western' and
do not always indicate relevant explanations for a set of circumstances that do not
often originate in a western context (Martin, 2006: 219).

The global perspectives that have resonance with a social justice perspective can
be seen to have a high degree of relevance. For example, anti-oppressive/anti-
discriminatory and feminist practices alert one to the use of power, the maintenance
of power and the importance of understanding resilience and perseverance within the
group being discussed. Galthung and Hoivik (1971) point to the need to explore

underpinning structural and cultural processes that contribute to structural violence. It is also important to deconstruct social practices as these are embedded in the social fabric and come together to form 'taken-for-granted' ways of operating.

On a national level, policies relating to inclusion and exclusion are very important. Vasta, (2004) and Papillion (2002), discuss the value and social capital that can be added to areas by embracing diversity and they regard the 'inclusion' of migrants and refugees as a way of developing 'cultural capital'. They recommend that the process of inclusion of the migrant is discussed at the settlement stage and includes the provision of appropriate and suitable housing, education and health. Papillion also talks about the necessary response of the 'local' with the state policies and procedures and the value of integration of specific Non-Government Organizations (NGOs) with government structures. Papillion's 'Key Dimensions of Sustainable Diversity and Inclusion' include a range of factors from skills training and educational programmes through to anti-discrimination measures in employment and housing. These theories interrogate racist attitudes and behaviours towards those who are 'excluded' (Papillion, 2002: 5).

At a professional practice level understandings about theories of grief and loss can be valuable to assist people to resolve their past experiences and progress to lead positive lives. The consideration of Eisenbruch's work is essential, as it discusses 'cultural bereavement', and reinforces the individual's cultural interpretation of their situation and ways of resolving it. He states: 'A comprehensive approach to the diagnosis of refugee mental health must be culturally relevant, assume nothing about distress versus disorder and allow for the patient's cultural constructions of mental health' (Eisenbruch, 1991: 678). These understandings of loss and grief discuss the often systematic and painful losses endured before people leave their home country and their absolute lack of choice about leaving their homeland (see Pedersen, 2002). This makes the structural violence experienced in their new country doubly pervasive and harmful for children and families.

Asylum seekers in the community: impact on children

Many families although afforded full refuge status, have to wait for long periods before being eligible to apply to become Australian citizens. During this period of uncertainty the major concerns raised about asylum seeker children primarily relate to health and education. It can also be maintained that their sense of identity and belonging is also hindered during this period.

A number of research studies indicate that children who are asylum seekers have a number of health related problems (Lynch and Cunninghame, 2000, Harris and Telfer, 2001; Davidson, Skull, Chaney, *et al.*, 2004). Prior to their arrival, the situation in their home country might have had an adverse effect on their health. However, once in Australia the child and their family may be denied access to universal health care, namely, Medicare. If the parents are prevented from working due to visa conditions then access to optical, dental and psychiatric services is extremely limited for the child (Correa-Velez, Gifford and Bice, 2005).

Another factor is the complexity, variation and difficulties associated with visas. Not all Temporary Protection Visa[1] holders have access to free medical services. Restrictions are also placed on benefits that asylum seeker families can claim in the United Kingdom (see de Albornoz, 2006).

With regard to mental health, there are concerns regarding the risks associated with imposing excessively hard conditions on asylum seekers. As a result of the trauma that families have experienced before arriving in the new country, including an often dangerous and distressing journey, adults and children are often vulnerable and lack the support to withstand the instability and anxiety that occurs when waiting for legal resolution of their citizenship status. Children are clearly caught up in family dilemmas – Silove, Steel, and Watters (2000) and Fazel and Stein (2002) point out that children are at greater risk of developing psychological problems.

Education is clearly of considerable significance to children of asylum seekers. The Children's Society (2003) has highlighted the important role that teachers and schools can play in enabling children to interact with other children and developing the necessary language and other skills to cope in the new environment. As Lynch (2004) has pointed out, this process can be impeded by continuing uncertainty about unresolved legal status. She noted that one child had been in Australia for eight years and still at 15 years of age, a permanent visa had not been obtained (Lynch, 2004). In another study, where 124 of 1,299 asylum seeking families living in Northern Sweden started to experience mental health problems, it is notable that almost every child's health condition improved when they gained permission to stay in Sweden (Joelsson and Dahlin, 2005).

Anderson (2001) draws attention to how children and families whose legal status remain unresolved as a result of uncertainty about whether they will have to return to their country of origin, find it difficult to develop a sense of belonging. Children can be caught trying both to 'belong' whilst also trying to stay close to old inherited associations. This can be painful and distressing for children and their parents (Anderson, 2001). Children without a clear sense of identity and belonging may not only experience personal distress but retrospectively view their childhood experiences as punitive, unnecessary and negating of their rights as children.

Mandatory detention: impact on children

Mandatory detention originated as part of the 1958 Migration Act and reflected a harsh political climate. It was implemented following the 1989 landing of a boat

---

1 Temporary Protection Visas are issued to asylum seekers and their families and some refugees in Australia. They are valid for 30 months and do not guarantee permanency. Some versions allow work, some do not; some versions allow access to medical services and associated services. But they vary considerably. (Australian Department of Immigration and Citizenship, Fact Sheet 67: Temporary Protection Visas)

from Indochina carrying twenty-six people, in a very remote part of Australia. According to Mares, it quickly became far more formalized with detention centres being built in other remote parts of Australia and being declared off-limits to journalists and NGOs. Whilst such courses of action have been contested and a number of appeals to the United Nations High Commissioner for Refugees (UNHCR) have been lodged about the inhumane treatment asylum seekers receive, the policy and practice has remained, albeit in a much moderated form (Mares, 2004; Wacogne, 2003). Now children are mostly not detained, as they are housed in community centres, but the impact of this policy on refugees and asylum seekers and on children has been profound. It is a policy of deterrence (Refugee Council of Australia, 2007).

For people in detention, there is evidence of increased despair and clinical depression among adults (Australian Council of Heads of Schools of Social Work, 2006). In a study conducted by Sultan and O'Sullivan, of the thirty-three adult detainees in a detention centre in Villawood, Sydney, very high numbers had sleep problems, regular nightmares, feelings of intense bitterness and chronic feelings of helplessness and depression. The writers also speak of difficulty with memory and concentration and of the increased likelihood of violence against the self (Sultan and O'Sullivan, 2001).

One of the major results of mandatory detention on children has been the deterioration of health, particularly mental health. In addition, they have limited access to medical, optical and dental services and they mostly are unable to go to school. They have had no confidence that they will not be deported and most importantly, they are unable to begin a settlement process with their new country. Combined with limited language and educational programmes, children who have been in detention often have serious developmental and educational delays (Cemlyn and Briskman, 2003: 171). Sultan and O'Sullivan state:

> The detention environment, exposure to actions such as hunger strikes, demonstrations, episodes of self-harm and suicide attempts, and forcible-removable procedures, all impact on a child's sense of security and stability. A secondary effect is mediated via the parents, whose ability to provide a caring and nurturing environment is progressively undermined.
>
> (Sultan and O'Sullivan, 2001: 596)

In detention families are excluded from everyday community interaction. As the majority of detention centres are located in remote areas, there is little community support available and the opportunity for emotional connections are limited. Political campaigns geared towards gaining votes by appealing to racist sentiments also influence public opinion about asylum seeker and promote stereotypical responses. This again can militate against the development of effective community support systems.

The United Kingdom provides another example of asylum seekers being used for purposes of political manipulation. Policies such as these clearly undermine the human rights of asylum seekers and their children.

Governments have persistently ignored the effects of their policies towards asylum seeker children and it is pertinent that Australia did not introduce changes in legislation to take children into account until 2005. However, asylum seeker children spend very long periods in community detention with all the associated ill-effects previously discussed. There has been a concerted and consistent effort by a number of groups to alert and influence the government about the humanitarian concerns for asylum seekers in detention. The overwhelming response has been that the importance of deterring people from entering the country without mandated documents, and the safety and protection of the country from suspected terrorists outweighs the needs of what are regarded in political terms as a relatively small group. Thus, asylum seeker children are caught between Australia's 'duty of care' to children, and political expediency.

Government responses can be seen as a form of structural violence. This is manifested in Australia's political history of non-acceptance of difference and its fear of losing its particular identity. Global concern about national security and fear about terrorism, fanned by sensational media reporting, have been used to legitimate government responses and the form of state violence alluded to in this chapter. Asylum seekers are not dependent people needing welfare services for long periods of time. Clearly they require employment, housing, healthcare and education. If these facilities are available then asylum seekers can make a significant contribution to their host country and have a 'better life'.

Implications for human service professionals

The most valuable role that human service professionals can play is in the role of advocacy. That children are no longer in detention in Australia is partly due to the strong advocacy efforts of individuals and groups. While it is important for human service professionals to offer a range of services, they also need to draw attention to the ways in which asylum seekers and their children are abused by the system.

There needs to be far more public debate about the issues facing asylum seekers, and human service professionals have a role to play in this debate (Refugee Council of Australia, 2007). This has national as well as international implications (Jones, 2001; Christie, 2003: 230).

With regard to education, many children and young people report the need for a positive construction of the asylum seeker in the school curriculum. Some of the negative attitudinal beliefs expressed can be addressed by the adoption of a proactive stance. In a twelve-week programme conducted in Canada, for example, it was found that creative workshops in the classroom can have a beneficial effect on the self-esteem and mental health of the children of asylum seekers from various cultures and backgrounds. As stated,

> The workshops participate in the reconstruction of a meaningful personal world while simultaneously strengthening the link of the child to the group. They also transform the teachers' perceptions of newcomers by placing an

emphasis on their strength and their resilience, while not negating their vulnerabilities.

(Rousseau, Drapeau, Lacroix, Bagilishya
and Heusch, 2005: 180)

This reinforces the need for inclusion of the issues of the children of asylum seekers in primary and secondary school curriculums.

In conclusion, a balanced multi-layered approach is necessary to contribute to change. Understanding the ways in which asylum seekers are subjected to political and media manipulation is an important step in recognizing their basic human rights and a need for sensitive support systems. National governments are clearly failing asylum seekers and are contravening their basic human rights internationally. Perhaps the only way forward is for there to be concerted action at an international level in relation to Article 14. Recognizing this perhaps, constitutes the only way of overcoming state violence towards this disparate and persistently disadvantaged group.

Chapter summary

Violence and the state: asylum seeker children

- Children, if not in detention, can be in detention-like settings (in the community, near the detention setting), while their family is in detention, with little access to appropriate schooling, health and other essential requirements.
- Children can be living in the community with varied access to free medical, dental and optometry services, dependent on their visa, which at best, offers temporary protection. Often they have problems that are caused by their history, but also as a result of their current situations.
- Children cannot have a sense of belonging with their new country, nor can they return to their country of origin. The despondency of children and young people to this political 'policy of deterrence', along with a passive acceptance by the mainstream population constitutes structural violence.
- The central focus of this chapter is Australia, as it is the only country that has detained asylum seeker families, including children, but there is evidence of 'policies of deterrence' in many other western countries.
- Strategies for helping services to address this population group are discussed, with the major strategy being advocacy at all levels of community and government to bring about some improvements for this vulnerable group in the community.

12 Out of the asylum

From restraints to freedom?

Zita Weber

'Forget it,' he said. 'You aren't going to lunch. You're going to the hospital.' He looked triumphant.

It was very quiet out in the suburbs before eight in the morning. And neither of us had anything more to say. I heard the taxi pulling up in the doctor's driveway.

He took me by the elbow – pinched me between his stout fingers – and steered me outside. Keeping hold of my arm, he opened the back door of the taxi and pushed me in. His big head was in the backseat with me for a moment. Then he slammed the door shut.

The driver rolled his window down halfway.

'Where to?'

Coatless in the chilly morning, planted on his sturdy legs in his driveway, the doctor lifted one arm to point at me.

'Take her to McLean,' he said, 'and don't let her out till you get there.'

I let my head fall back against the seat and shut my eyes. I was glad to be riding in a taxi instead of having to wait for the train.

(Kaysen, 2000: 8–9)

Echoes of the past

Susanna Kaysen's narrative account of being put in a taxi and sent to McLean Hospital after one session with a psychiatrist she'd never seen before epitomizes what could routinely happen in 1967. Boston's McLean, affiliated with Harvard Medical School, is a psychiatric hospital renowned for its famous clientele – Sylvia Plath, who is said to have captured some memories of her time spent within McLean's walls in *The Bell Jar*, Robert Lowell, James Taylor, Anne Sexton and Ray Charles. Over the years, McLean had developed arguably a glamorous reputation – for a psychiatric hospital. But Susanna Kaysen's lived experience, or what Beresford (2004) calls, 'experiential knowledge', at McLean both presented and challenged the management of mental distress, the infringement of individual liberty, the validity of compulsory treatment and other forms of coercion.

Writing thirty-eight years later, Bracken and Thomas said, 'Many service users find the process of psychiatric assessment painful and sometimes oppressive' (2005: 123). The oppressive nature of assessment and subsequent treatment these authors suggest, is related to how the professional's gaze does not seek to interpret or to understand, but merely to identify and describe. In Kaysen's account, as in many others, the professionals in charge of her care made no attempt to enter her mental world, nor to understand her lived reality. As Bracken and Thomas suggest, such separation of the lived experience from the naming of the entity or syndrome stems from a modernist framework in which phenomenology involves a 'search for knowledge about "the other"' (2005: 123) without an attempt to grasp the human reality of the experience presented by the individual. Manning (1998) has critiqued the professional task of defining the nature of the consumer and what the consumer needs. Segal, Silverman and Temkin (1993) identified how a diagnosis could become a form of identity. Susanna Kaysen, the depressive.

This chapter will explore the rise of the phenomenon of the contemporary collective movement of consumers of mental health services and its importance in challenging the history of past institutional and professional violence, abuse and oppression. Goffman (1961) described psychiatric hospitals as total institutions that lead to apathy, passivity and resignation among patients. Based on her own and others' experiences of being hospitalized, Judi Chamberlin (1978) reached a similar conclusion that psychiatric hospitals promote weakness and dependency and powerlessness.

Over the past few decades, the emphasis has shifted to focusing on helping the individual remain in their community environment and to issues related to social justice and equality. There are many stories that can be told about the rise of the consumer movement from the earliest recorded collective action, the 'Petition of the Poor Distracted People in the House of Bedlam' in 1620 (Barnes, 2002); however, what makes the development of this general movement interesting is the importance and centrality of the contemporary consumer voice. Barnes points to the 'insertion of service users into spaces and places that would have been unimaginable in the 1970s' (2002: 3). Consumers and consumer advocates can now sit on advisory committees, offer training and consultation to human service professionals and professionals within the mental health care system have come out as service users and been able to draw on and share experiences with peers.

Nevertheless, there is room for further critiquing of the dominant concepts in mental health and theories around distress and models of helping based on the lived experience of consumers that might be of use to professionals (Campbell, 2002; Wallcraft and Michaelson, 2002). Both negative and positive perspectives have been forwarded by individual consumers and woven into the grand narrative about the violence, abuse and oppression experienced by consumers within the mental health services. Bassman posits that for too long, mental health consumers had been disenfranchised. He advocates that consumers challenge the past realities of the 'medically based drug-dominated oppressive mental health system'

(Bassman, 2001: 31) as well as challenge current beliefs about whose reality is privileged in the narrative of mental health service delivery. Issues related to power and stigma and their oppressive effects on consumers will be explored against the backdrop of the promises and challenges that contemporary mental health services face in the wake of previous generations of abuse, violence, oppression and very often, neglect of the 'patients' within the care of the system. The movement towards building partnerships between consumers and professionals and the unwritten charter of becoming allies in emancipation will be offered in an attempt to capture the spirit of contemporary endeavours.

Promises and challenges

It might be argued that at the beginning of the twenty-first century, the management of mental illness and mental distress remains a contestable arena and that policies and practices have not sustained the momentum for reform that had been set with the movement in the 1970s toward deinsitutionalization and community care (Meadows, Singh and Grigg, 2007; Pilgrim and Hitchman, 1999). In this post-institutional stage, mental health delivery and practice has been confronted by 'consumerism' and the question of citizenship of people formerly called 'patients' (Pilgrim and Hitchman, 1999). Oliver (1996) writing about disability generally, articulates the point that the contemporary context demands reconceptualizing the problem – from needs to rights. Consequent to these trends, shifts in accountability and involvement by the different players in the system have meant that people experiencing mental illness are now more visible and audible and that service providers are required to be more accountable for their actions, more willing to challenge services that are disabling, redress environments that are restrictive and reflect upon practices that are discriminatory and exclusionary (Chamberlin, 1990; Fawcett and Karban, 2005; Hudson, 1999; M. Oliver, 1996). Self-advocacy has become a significant positive belief and practice amongst consumers, recognizing the possibility and desirability of people speaking out and acting for themselves (Campbell, 2002). For instance, in the United Kingdom, Survivors Speak Out was founded in 1986 as a national networking organization promoting the idea and practice of self-advocacy.

What is uncontestable is that, in the last quarter of the twentieth century and the beginning of the twenty-first century, there has been ever increasing awareness of the need for policy reform, developing better daily practices and conducting research that reflects the experiences of all the players in the mental health arena: or professionals and consumers (Bassman, 2001; Burstow, 2004; Jacobson and Curtis, 2000; Nelson, 1994).

Fighting oppression and the power of pejorative language

In the decades since the 1970s, the words and language of people who would come to call themselves variously consumers/users/survivors/ex-patients, have become more forceful and their voices much louder. In the United States, the term 'c/s/x' refers to the coalitional nature of the group – consumers/survivors/ ex-patients, with many differences between them. For instance, those people who totally reject psychiatry identify as 'ex-patients', those who are critical consumers refer to themselves as 'consumers' and those who are somewhere in between identify as 'survivors'. These words provide people with new identity positions (Morrison, 2005). What all three groups have in common, is their struggle with and resistance to mainstream psychiatry's core individualizing and pathologizing convictions (Lewis, 2006). C/s/x members and those who support them, 'talk back' (Morrison, 2005) to psychiatry, both individually and collectively. The people who identify with any of these groups refuse the passive 'patient' role in favour of 'resistant identities' (Morrison, 2005).

In the United States in the 1980s and 1990s, the consumer movement worked to change the language that defined them. Many consumers objected to the term 'chronic' which implies irreversibility and poor prognosis (Bachrach, 1988; Hatfield and Lefley, 1993). In recognition of this, the National Institute of Mental Health began substituting terms such as 'seriously and persistently' and even 'severely mentally ill' (Hatfield and Lefley, 1993). However, some consumers prefer the term 'psychiatrically disabled' to 'mentally ill'. Other consumers have resented being identified with labels that begin with the definite article 'the' – and with specific acronyms (Hatfield and Lefley, 1993). These consumers argue that they are stripped of their individual identity when they are designated as belonging to a group of people who are 'the CMI' (chronically mentally ill) or 'the SMI' (seriously mentally ill). Making this point clearly, one consumer has suggested: 'If we can be called CMIs – the chronically mentally ill – then they, the mental health professionals, can be called MHPs. If we must be relegated to a three-letter acronym – and basically stripped of our identity and individuality – then they too can be lumped into one pot' (Blaska, 1991: 173).

In the United Kingdom, language generally has become more inclusive and terminology has shifted from 'psychiatric' to 'mental health' (Fawcett and Karban, 2005) when describing the professional task and the services offered and the term 'mental distress' has found favour amongst service users (Rogers and Pilgrim, 1993, 2001). Attention also has been given to nomenclature, with changes such as the expression 'a person being a schizophrenic' to 'a person living with schizophrenia'. Such shifts in language signal a move to a more respectful attitude towards those people living with mental illness.

In the Editor's choice segment in the *British Medical Journal* ("The Editor's Choice", 30 November 2002), quoting research by Simpson and House (2002), the opinion was forwarded that involving users or consumers in delivering mental health services is effective and that the policy in the NHS (National Health Service in the United Kingdom) to ensure that consumers are present whenever important decisions are being made about the service is encapsulated in the 'Nothing about me without me' slogan.

Nevertheless, along with some innovative changes have been an equal number of challenges, as people formerly called patients continue their campaign to have their voices heard to have their narratives taken seriously, to influence the policy environment and direction and to become more involved in research. Points of resistance and challenge remain as consumers lobby and advocate for improvements and change in the belief that 'the political is the personal' as much as 'the personal is the political' (Watson and Williams, 1992). Wappett (2002) points out that the key components of the women's movement are generalizable to the disability rights and self-determination movements. These three key components are: (1) the need to unify academic theory that can drive the movement; (2) creating groups at local, state and national levels to seek opportunities for consciousness, spur self-advocacy and motivate political action; and (3) aggressive political action at all levels of government to ensure that demands are heard.

In the United Kingdom, 'psychiatric survivors' have formed social movements and in North America, consumers have drawn attention to their agenda at forums such as Psychiatry Survivor Pride Day. In March 2000, Support Coalition International (a worldwide coalition of psychiatric survivor groups) held an historic international conference in Knoxville, Tennessee, attended by thousands of representatives. Subsequently, a statement, a 'Call to Action' was issued:

> We call upon all people committed to human rights to organize and fight against the passage and implementation of legislation making it easier to lock up and forcibly drug people labeled with psychiatric disorders, legislation that is creating the backwardness of the twenty-first century not just in back wards but also in our homes. We call upon all people committed to human rights to work together to build a mental health system that is based upon the principle of self-determination on a belief in our ability to recover, and on our right to define what recovery is and how best to achieve it. We call upon all people who have used mental health services to heal each other by telling our stories. We call for the creation of literature and other arts that use our truth to educate, to inform, and to validate our culture and our experience. We call upon elected officials, political candidates, and those with power over our lives to recognize and honor the legitimacy of our concerns through their policy statements, legislative proposals, and in their actions; and we hereby give notice that we will do whatever it takes to ensure that we are heard, that our rights are protected, and that we can live freely and peacefully in our communities.
>
> (Support Coalition International, 2000: 5)

Essentially, this statement declares a commitment to human rights, humanistic values and social justice; asserts agency and announces an intention to work towards change; invites service providers with power to hear and to act and it highlights the importance of recovery.

The balance of power

Many narrative accounts over the decades have evocatively captured practices and the harsh policies from the past: the routine nature of involuntary admission, lack of informed consent, professional abuse of power, oppression of the 'patient's' rights to self-direction and self-determination (McLean, 2003; McNeill, 1998; Millett, 1974; Sutherland, 1976). Such narrative accounts tell of experiences in which these narrators were acted upon by 'expert' others and where there was scant recognition of the 'subjective' experience of the distressed person. Olsen and Epstein (2001) comment on such past practices as the 'objectification' of the 'patient' often leading to a situation in which explanations and information regarding diagnosis and treatment were not considered important. When authority is vested in only the professional in the relationship, a dynamic in which that person has 'power over' the consumer develops (Segal et al., 1993).

We might be lulled into thinking that the bad old days when doctors (and other health professionals) were dominant and 'patients' were expected to be patient and powerless are over. We might believe that practices expecting compliance by consumers are only distant memories. As a young social work student on placement in an admission ward in a major psychiatric centre in Sydney in the early 1970s I heard complaints by staff daily about 'non-compliant patients' and witnessed the punishments meted out. I also sat with patients and heard them talk about their sense of powerlessness, feelings of oppression and hopelessness in being in a drugged state against their will and 'specialled' to wear pyjamas. Some of them even named certain practices, such as ECT (electro convulsive therapy), as violent and inhumane. Notions of rights, self-determination and self-empowerment were hinted at, sometimes named in lay words and language by the patients. But in the institution in which they were hospitalized, they were the least powerful players.

Kaysen's narrative is embedded in a time when the dominant social narrative of people with mental health problems labelled them as dangerous 'psychos' (Rappaport, 1993, 1995). Such accounts give an insight into the power imbalances and the dynamics that, it has been argued, constrained mental health and contributed to hindering mental health improvements (Burstow and Weitz, 1988). Whilst deinstitutionalization and community care have become common practices in many parts of the world, in Hungary, for instance, many people with mental illness still live in large institutions called 'psychiatric homes' or 'psychiatric rehabilitation homes' (Weber and Bugarszki, 2007).

The many personal narratives that have emerged in the last decade are not all negative. Diverse opinions are expressed in an anthology, *Speaking Our Minds* (Read and Reynolds, 1996). What these narratives highlight is the many different ways in which people interpret their experiences and the importance of context and meaning when exploring mental distress and the role of power and control in mental health services (Bracken and Thomas, 2005).

Olsen and Epstein comment, 'The kinds of power relationships that operate within the mental health field are largely (still) constructed through institutions of social control. This means that the "balances of power" in this field become entrenched, fixed, and resistant to change' (2001: 9). The psychiatrist Ron Leifer participated in the Foucault Tribunal, a mock trial organized by the psychiatric survivor movement in Germany in 1998. In his subsequent critique of psychiatry, Leifer (2000) invites a dialogue and argues for new paradigms for understanding human behaviour and mental distress, claiming that the medical model discourse and the context in which mental health services are delivered enable and justify an extra-legal, covert form of social control over the lives of people with mental illness. Insofar as people with a mental illness are considered not responsible for themselves, the medical model allows for the violation of human rights.

Susanna Kaysen's narrative account highlights the roles clearly: the doctor as the 'expert helper' and Susanna Kaysen as the 'inadequate help receiver', which in turn, created a difference in status and self-esteem and thus a difference in power (Boltz, 1992; Segal et al., 1993). Zussman's (1992) observations about 'the impersonality of medicine' and a lack of 'orientation to the patient as a person' were to profoundly affect the personal and political power of people with mental disabilities until their voices were brought to the fore with the rise of the consumer movement. Chamberlin, a former 'patient' and a long-time activist, has written extensively about experiences of oppression and exclusion and how 'the mad themselves have remained largely voiceless' (1990: 323).

In the early 1960s, the anti-psychiatry movement, most identified with Thomas Szasz (1961) and R.D. Laing (1965), had started to challenge the medical model of mental health that was used to legitimate coercive psychiatric interventions, although even within that movement, there was evidence of benign paternalism. The self-proclaimed 'expert' had the power to interpret the distressed individual's lived experience (Clarke, 2004; Hopton, 2006), in what were called 'therapeutic communities'. These communities ostensibly offered democratic living arrangements in alternative settings where people were free from treatment and where doors were unlocked and residents did not see their doctors and nurses as gaolers. It was thought that real therapy could be offered in such an environment and the open doors would respect patients as persons.

What effect has opening the doors permanently and offering community care had on the lives of those people living with a mental illness?

Change of heart or change of concept?

Deinstitutionalization and with it the opening of doors into the community, promised to uncover the real illness, uncomplicated by confinement, frustration and resentment which previously locked up patients had experienced (Clarke, 2004). With the development of community-based long-term services and opportunities and policy and attitudinal advancements have come the possibilities and challenges of self-determination and the expression of the hope for full citizenship for those people living with mental illness and mental distress (Powers, Ward, Ferris, et al., 2002). The rise of a movement around empowerment, self-advocacy and the call for person-directed services is far removed from Susanna Kaysen's experience.

In 1999 in the United States, a National Summit on Self-Determination and Consumer-Direction was held, and the self-determination movement acknowledged its roots in the human and civil rights movement. The principles of self-determination that came from this event were enshrined in a living document that nominates the principles of: freedom for people living with disabilities to determine for themselves what is important in their lives; authority to determine and direct their lives, including controlling their money, voting and entering into contractual arrangements, such as buying a home, getting married; support to meaningfully participate in their communities, to identify life goals and to have access to a life with opportunities and potential; and responsibility, insofar as having the ordinary obligations of citizenship like other members of the community (Alliance for Self-Determination, 2001).

The emerging concepts of consumer direction and consumer choice have highlighted the issues related to citizenship and community care models in which informed consent and the right to refuse care feature (Batavia, 2002). In a landmark court decision in the United State's Supreme Court ruled that unjustified institutionalization constitutes discrimination under the Americans with Disabilities Act of 1990 and that individuals must be provided with care in the most integrated setting appropriate to the individual's home and community (Olmstead, 1999). The Mental Health Act (1990) in New South Wales (NSW) Australia, puts forward the notion of least restrictive alternatives, based on the belief that the dignity and the freedom of individuals is important and that government control needs limiting (Cocks, 1989). People have the right to the least restrictive care and should not be hospitalized if they can be cared for in the community.

Personal motivation, self-direction and self-determination are all difficult to realize in the face of internalized powerlessness or oppression (Lerner, 1991; Rose and Black, 1985, 1990). Many people living with mental illness experience multiple oppression. Gender has significance when considering the lives of many women whose experiences also are shaped by racism (Bayne Smith, 1996; Cook and Watt, 1992; Holland, 1995; Ismail, 1996), classism (Bayne Smith, 1996; G.W. Brown and Harris, 1978), homophobia (Bridget and Lucille, 1996; L.S. Brown, 1996; Herek and Berril, 1990) and ageism (Nadien, 1996; Padgett, Burns and Grau, 1998). Many studies (Beckwith, 1993; Broverman, Broverman, Clarkson, Rosenkrantz and Vogel, 1970; Kaplan, 1983) as well as historical analyses (Busfield, 1996; Fernando, Ndegwa and Wilson, 1998; Russell, 1995; Ussher, 1991) have shown that women's feelings, thoughts and behaviours are more likely to be defined as 'mad' than those of men and that historically, psychiatry has had an enthusiasm for labelling experiences and behaviour of oppressed people as disturbed and disordered.

The literature on men's mental health is comparatively slight, although the over-representation of African Caribbean men in the United Kingdom and Indigenous men in Australia in statistics relating to compulsory admissions is well documented (Burgmann, 2003; Healthcare Commission, 2005). However, some researchers have traced important links between social inequalities and men's mental health. Baker-Miller (1976), Collins (1998), Miller and Bell (1996) and Thomas (1996) have all argued that the privileged male role imposes expectations about masculinity that may have a detrimental effect on the mental health of men and the women and children in their families. Many men experience the oppression of bullying, brutality, sexual abuse and violence within their home and in their communities; however, these traumas are under-reported because of the injunctions placed on emotional entitlement – real men shouldn't have let these events happen, or shouldn't let them matter (Freeman and Fallot, 1997; Miller and Bell, 1996).

Honouring of stories of consumers/survivors/ex-patients and respecting the power of an insider's knowledge of what it's like, what's been experienced in terms of help and support – and what was done in the name of treatment – has become accepted practice. Too often in the past as Ronald Bassman, himself a psychologist and psychiatric survivor, comments, the manner in which services were extended meant they were 'to and for but rarely with – those lacking the power or voice to fight the abuses and keep their basic human rights' (2001: 34).

Compelling treatments without hospitalization and the need for coercion remain in many countries committed to deinstitutionalization, as the general public are persuaded that community care works to manage people with mental health problems. Rogers and Pilgrim (2001) challenge the widely held view regarding the demise of institutional psychiatry. In Britain, for instance, they point to the emphasis on risk and safety issues in recent mental health policy. In Australia, similar legislation, with coercion and control at its core has been enacted in some states. According to Rogers and Pilgrim (2001), little has changed during the past hundred years. Psychiatry still has control of the mental health agenda in terms of control, coercion and exclusion. They extend their argument to challenge the notion that the consumer-led movement has made the impact some would claim. It is their contention that in spite of such trends, contemporary mental health practice is allied to biological approaches and that coercion continues to be the primary focus of the whole mental health system. Lewis (2006) and Morrison (2005) have forwarded a similar argument, adding that the 'neurochemical self' is in danger of eclipsing the real selves of consumers. Nevertheless, consumer activists continue to work towards creating a world that understands and embraces psychic difference and to challenge a world that all too often responds with 'psychiatric labeling, forced treatment and dehumanization' (Morrison, 2005: 215).

Stigma and internalized oppression

Labels can stigmatize and terms such as 'chronic' can increase the stigma. Labels can also promote distancing behaviour in professionals (Gutierree, Parsons and Cox, 1998). This is well illustrated by a social work author, Anonymous, who challenged the stigma of her label when, 'I do not reveal my past diagnostic status at employment interviews ... Would you have a "chronic schizophrenic-undifferentiated" for anything more than sanding furniture or sorting screws?' (1990: 391).

Sartorius (1999) claimed that one of the last obstacles to better mental health care was the still present, ubiquitous and in his view, growing stigma of mental illness. Stigma occurs when a label represents a perceived deviation from expected behaviour. In some societies, it can lead to positive discrimination, for instance, if the symptoms of the mental illness are interpreted as being an indication of a divine possession of the person. Mostly, however, stigma results in a negative discrimination of the person. Stigma and the intolerance of difference can be particularly pervasive in rural areas (Manning, Zibalese-Crawford and Downey, 1994). People may internalize these norms and stereotypes (Boltz, 1992; Chamberlin, 1990; Manning, 1998). This internalized oppression can manifest as experiences of shame, lowered expectations of themselves and fears of rejection (Boltz, 1992; Manning, Zibalese-Crawford and Downey, 1994). As one person explained, 'We stigmatize ourselves through denial, lack of acceptance, language and isolation. … We picked up the language of the professionals and use it to stigmatize each other' (Manning et al., 1994: 8).

According to the World Health Organization (WHO), 450 million people worldwide are affected by mental distress (WHO, Mental Health Denied Citizens). WHO identifies mental health problems in terms of the undefined and hidden burdens. One of the nominated hidden burdens is stigma (WHO, November 2001).

The World Psychiatric Association (WPA) has initiated an international programme to fight the stigma and discrimination associated with schizophrenia and since its inception in 1996, more than twenty countries, including Spain, Austria, Germany, Poland, Greece, Italy, Turkey, Slovakia, Brazil, Egypt, Morocco, Chile, India and Romania have signed up to implement anti-stigma programmes. The United Kingdom, Australia and the United States and Canada, took part in this global drive and in these countries campaigns against stigma have been undertaken by governments and non-government organizations over the past two decades.

The WPA has estimated that the participating countries have undertaken approximately 200 anti-stigma interventions. These interventions were 'directed towards well-defined target groups in an effort to address different parts of the vicious cycles that lead to discrimination and prejudice' (Sartorius and Schulz, 2005: xvi). For instance, in the United Kingdom, workshops were implemented with police officers and in schools. Other anti-discrimination campaigns have been sponsored by the National Institute for Mental Health in England (www. mindout.net) and the Royal College of Psychiatrists (www.changingminds. co.uk). In Australia, the WPA global programme has worked in partnership with SANE Australia (www.sane.org) to develop information resources for the media as well as for those living with mental illness, their families and caregivers. This partnership has achieved significant success in working in collaboration with the media to resource them with information that supports the demystifying and destigmatizing of images and language and impresses upon the media the effects of negative media portrayals on those living with mental illness. In Denver, Colorado, anti-stigma groups have been conducted within the criminal justice system to help reduce fear of the mentally ill and to ensure that police officers, probation officers, corrections officers, attorneys and judges all have a better understanding of the lived experience of consumers with a mental illness. In September 1997, the WPA held a press conference during a meeting of the Canadian Psychiatric Association in Calgary, Alberta, Canada. At the press event to announce that Calgary would be the pilot site for the global programme to fight stigma and discrimination, a young woman called Michelle Miserelli stepped forward and introduced herself as a consumer and a mother who had been invited to speak about the challenges first hand. For some of the journalists present, what Michelle Miserelli had to say was not only powerful and moving, but also marked the first time they had heard an individual speaking about their experience and describing the discrimination she faced (Sartorius and Schulz, 2005).

Towards progressive mental health policy

Over the past decade, in Britain, North America and Australia, there has been increasing public pressure for governments to respond to the perceived deficits in service delivery within the mental health arena. It seems that Cinderella might finally be going to the ball. One case manager in a Melbourne-based, Australian mental health community service commented,

> So much is changing, and not before time. Ideas about social inclusion, self-determination, recovery, and consumer rights all have powerful implications for policies that some consumers believe are still severely limiting people's rights to truly determine what happens in their lives. Recent government initiatives, at federal and state levels are reflecting a more holistic conception of mental illness – a more inclusive view of the person with the mental illness. National Mental Health Practice Standards, for example, bring home the fact that consumers and carers count, their thoughts and feelings do matter. Sometimes it takes a document and some push to implement it, before policies are taken on board at the coal-face.
>
> (Weber, 2005, unpublished)

In 2002 in Australia, the *National Practice Standards for the Mental Health Workforce* was released and of the twelve standards nominated, Standard 2 refers to 'Consumer and carer participation'. This practice standard entreats professionals to encourage and support the participation of consumers and carers in determining their individual treatment and care, as well as requiring professionals to actively 'promote, encourage and support the participation of consumers, family members and/or carers in the planning, implementation and evaluation of mental health service delivery' (p. xi). As Fawcett and Karban state, 'The National Standard for the Mental Health Services have been presented in Australia as reflecting a strong commitment to values related to human rights, dignity and empowerment' (2005: 58).

In the United Kingdom, the incoming Labour government of 1997 highlighted the urgent need to 'modernize' the context and delivery of mental health services.

Since that time, several government policy documents have been forwarded, including *The National Service Framework for Mental Health* (Department of Health, 1999), which aims to improve health and social care by introducing service performance monitoring in seven nominated key areas (Fawcett and Karban, 2005). Other policy documents, for instance, *Inside/Outside* (Department of Health, 2003a) and *Delivering Race Equality: A Framework for Action* (Department of Health, 2003b) have highlighted specific issues such as the over-representation of certain minority ethnic groups in mental health services and the need to give specific attention to this area (Fawcett and Karban, 2005).

According to Duggan, Cooper and Foster, policy initiatives suffer from the fundamental difficulty of 'relating macro to micro preoccupations' (2002: 3). They comment that there is an absence of real people and evidence of 'a grasp of the lived experience of patients, carers or even professionals' in the policy documents and the thinking behind them. Nevertheless, recent trends have demonstrated that there is a dawning awareness that policy and practice need to be ever more closely intertwined. In 2006 in Australia, NSW Health, the state government responsible for delivering mental health services, issued a report – *A statewide approach to measuring and responding to consumer perceptions and experiences of adult mental health services.* Recommendations of this report would guide future directions in understanding and improving service quality. It was stated specifically that the report was about 'People who use mental health services (consumers) in NSW giving their feedback to services, and services and consumers working together to create a better mental health service' (2006: 4).

Building partnerships: becoming allies in emancipation

Given the history to date, the question becomes: how can we achieve effective and emancipatory services in the mental health arena? Becoming allies, forming partnerships between consumers and service providers, drawing on the ideas that emerge from a strengths-based perspective (Saleebey, 1992, 1996) and the development and application of notions of recovery (Harding and Zahniser, 1994; Harrison, Craig, Laska, et al., 2001), appears to be the way forward (Munford and Sanders, 1999; Sullivan and Munford, 2005). Bassman (2001) and Burstow (2004) have urged practitioners to familiarize themselves with and use the knowledge gained from the narratives and literature generated by consumers to draw on as appropriate. Many of these narratives reveal what Goffman (1963) called 'the spoiled identity', with which psychiatry and its practices left those exposed to the system. The consumer movement, in broad terms, works towards putting consumers on a path to acceptance and recovery with a renewed sense of self, and a positive identity.

Fawcett and Karban point out that the notion of recovery and the application of the social model of disability to inform mental health practice have lost some of their currency. As such ideas, with their potential for innovation become incorporated into policy, often the 'power of the original' (2005: 75) concept as defined by individual consumers is lost in the translation into policy documents. Jacobson and Curtis echo this sentiment and warn that consumer advocates have expressed concern that the recovery model might be a passing fashion and 'become little more than a new label on an old bottle simply another name for professional driven rehabilitation services (2000: 339). If recovery is to be a viable phenomenon for consumers then re-conceptualizing the relationship between the individual and the system is critical. If this is not done, as Jacobsen and Curtis say, 'we risk promulgating a cosmetic initiative that maintains the dependence of individuals on the system' (2000: 339).

Reporting on the Mind Freedom International Oral History Project, Cohen (2005), a leader in the international c/s/x movement, says that the project's research interviews highlighted the theme that people do not 'get better' or 'recover' until they take control of their lives: their 'treatment', whether it was medication, meditation, exercise or peer and social support.

It would be difficult to underestimate the profound challenges associated with successful community living for people with serious mental illness. The development of natural supports within the wider community setting is among the critical needs of people living with mental illness. One social worker, who works as a case manager in a Sydney-based community mental health service commented:

> The important thing is to make sure that we get our people integrated into real community activities and interacting with a cross-section of the population. For example, if someone wants to play football, it would be easy to form a team with just our own consumers. But that wouldn't be real. Ideally, I'd work towards helping him join a football team out in the community.
>
> (Weber, 2005, unpublished)

According to Hardiman (2004), the complex challenge for service providers is to assist consumers in genuine community transition, and to work towards minimizing the possibilities of social isolation and dependence on the mental health system. If independent living in the least restrictive manner is the goal, as it is in most Australian state legislation for instance, then the essential element of social support needs careful consideration. Without social support, independent living can become a misnomer, and seriously undermine a consumer's ability to exercise choice, be engaged with the wider community, and not remain reliant on the mental health system.

By working together to maximize community integration, consumers and service providers need to create what Simpson, Hornby, Davis and Murray (2005) have called emancipatory partnerships. They promote the idea that in order to sustain positive relationships with consumers and their families and carers, professionals need to adopt an attitude of openness, humility and belief that such a way of working together is the key to effective practice. They stress the need for such partnerships to be based on mutual respect, with the consumers and their families and carers valued for their expertise and considered the real experts regarding their experiences and lives. It follows that there must be open and clear two-way communication between consumers and professionals.

Implications for human service professionals

In a brief narrative piece, Irene Oliver, a social work practitioner, talks about how being a 'closet mental health consumer and service provider' has provided her with a unique perspective on the incongruity between what should and does happen sometimes when it comes to notions of partnerships and a respectful attitude towards consumers by professionals. She writes,

> Case managers who deride their clients behind their backs kid themselves if they think it does not show in their work. It does, one way or another, often not only to the detriment of the person with mental illness, but in increased tension with clients, decreased job satisfaction, and eventual staff burnout. Mental health professionals usually refuse to acknowledge their part in the supposedly therapeutic relationship. Clients are blamed for any problems that arise in case management. For many, the cycle of abuse continues within the mental health system.
>
> (Oliver, 2001: 139)

Unless service providers are vigilant about not taking over, they will inevitably start to take over (Bassman, 2001; Burstow, 2004; Chamberlin, 1978). Consumers acting as advisers and consultants, as advocates and educators as well as researchers and evaluators (Bassman, 2001; Beresford, 2004; Fawcett and Karban, 2005; Manning, 1998; Nelson, 1994; Nelson, Ochocka, Griffin and Lord, 1998; Pilgrim and Hitchman, 1999) has meant that services have been challenged, improved and shifts have occurred in the way professionals and consumers work together. Consultation and collaboration have become popular words used in relation to both policy and practice contexts. Collaborations should be just that – joint work towards a stated goal and a commitment to ongoing vigilance is essential. Nevertheless, Barnes and Bowl (2001) and Fawcett and Karban (2005) continue to caution about the tension between the power held by professionals and the challenges in any partnership with consumers whose experiences of both their mental distress and the service delivery system may be at odds with those of the professionals, or indeed, of the systemic notions of partnerships.

If collaboration is to become a reality, then what Peter Hulme (1996) calls 'collaborative conversations' between consumers and professionals need to take place. More fundamentally however, the marginalization and oppression that generations of consumers have experienced needs to be heard and redressed. In a submission to the Human Rights and Equal Opportunity Commission, formalized in the Burdekin Report (1993) the words of one consumer highlight the critical starting point for a future only dreamed of by Susanna Kaysen and others of her generation:

To speak for ourselves, [is] a basic human right. That it would be too stressful used to be the common rationalisation for our exclusion from the debates that affected our lives. Repression, misinterpretation and reinterpretation of one's reality is stressful.

(Submission No. 239, p. 3, 1993 as quoted in The Burdekin Report)

Susanna Kaysen probably would agree.

Chapter summary

Out of the asylum: from restraints to freedom?

- Over the past two decades, mental health consumers have raised their voices and demanded to be heard regarding the violence, abuse, oppression and neglect that they perceive to have been perpetrated on generations of 'patients'.
- Individual consumer narratives as well as collective consumer narratives have helped shape the consumer movement, which continues to challenge the power of the 'professional gaze' and to work towards self-determination and self-defined recovery.
- The contemporary consumer movement, the World Health Organization (WHO), and many national psychiatric bodies continue to work towards lessening stigma and the sense of oppression and 'surplus powerlessness' that consumers experience in the face of formal labels, adverse media portrayals and lingering wider community suspicion of those people living with mental illness.
- Together with the consumer movement lobby, increasing public and professional pressure for governments to respond to the perceived deficits in service delivery has resulted in renewed efforts to draft policy that is more inclusive and progressive.
- Policy stating standards and outcomes for mental health service delivery has created opportunities for more consultation and communication and an organizational culture that fosters the notion of building partnerships and consumers together with professionals, becoming allies in emancipation.

13 Violence against the self

Self-harm and suicide

Agi O'Hara

In this chapter, suicide is regarded as violence against the self and it is accepted that an individual may be prompted to take this course of action as a result of organizational, individual and/or routinized acts of abuse and oppression. As part of an exploration of this sensitive, yet sensational area, the various understandings of violence against the self or suicide will be explored. This will include an examination of the connections that can be made with 'self-harm' and an appraisal of motivational aspects and 'risk' factors. Policy factors will also be considered and the implications of self-inflicted violence for human service professionals will be discussed.

The theory developed by the nineteenth-century French sociologist Emile Durkheim, still influences present understandings about suicide or violence against the self. Durkheim identified various types of suicide, focusing particularly on the nature of the relationship between the suicidal person and their society (Shneidman and Mandelkorn, 1994). Durkheim differentiated between 'altruistic' suicide in which the person is culturally mandated to take their life as a means of maintaining their honour (for example, Japanese men committing hara-kiri, Hindu widows cremating themselves on their husband's funeral pyre); 'egoistic' suicide when the individual has 'too few ties with [their] community' (Shneidman and Mandelkorn, 1994: 89) and 'anomic' suicides when significant relationships have been suddenly disrupted (Shneidman and Mandelkorn, 1994). According to Durkheim (1952), the nature of the relationship between the suicidal person and their society is determined in part by the person's perception of their autonomy, sense of empowerment, their potential to control or influence significant events in their life and the nature and extent of connectedness of the relationships in which they are involved. As a result, experiences of oppression, disempowerment, disconnectedness, physical and psychological abuse, or violence in any form can be associated with violence against the self. The discussion to follow will primarily explore psychological factors, but will also make connections with those social forces which make the taking of violent action against the self more likely.

In the past, psychological theories generally focused on the various psychological disturbances that appeared to lead to violence against the self. However, more recently there have been significant advances in knowledge regarding specific types of experiences and issues that may enhance the likelihood of such violence. Numerous myths and unhelpful attitudes have been exposed that previously may have contributed to, or exacerbated violent acts against the self. Theorists worldwide have explored the relevance of many potentially contributing factors to the development of this form of violence with varying degrees of success. Some of the factors being explored include the interplay of genetic and environmental factors, the role of childhood and family adversities, familial transmission of violence against the self, the effects of gender role and sexual orientation, seasonal effects, rural versus urban pressures, unemployment, and the overall experience of power imbalances with the concomitant generation of various forms of discrimination, oppression and abuse.

Self-harm

The term deliberate self-harm (DSH) has been used to describe a range of behaviours such as cutting, picking at skin, self-poisoning, hair pulling, burning, abusing drugs or ingesting a non-ingestible substance, with the intention of causing self-harm. Deliberate self-harm is generally taken to relate to an outward expression of inner distress. It is seen to occur most frequently where an individual is not able to communicate through other means and it is notable that it can also be utilized as a means of self-soothing (Fox and Hawton, 2004). Deliberate self-harm in England and Wales, for example, accounts for over 100,000 accident and emergency attendances and admissions, each year (Poustie and Neville, 2004). It is more frequently exhibited in younger people and accounts for 'approximately 10 per cent of all hospitalisations of young people aged 15 to 19 in New Zealand' (Royal Australian and New Zealand College of Psychiatrists, 2005: 4), with females being more likely to engage in self-harm than males.

Due to the variety of self-harming behaviours and their sometimes unexpected outcomes, it can be difficult to differentiate between levels of lethality, that is the measure of probability that the behaviour will result in death or serious injury (Appleby, 1995). De Leo and Heller (2004) advocate focusing on motivation or intention when attempting to gain an understanding of the prevalence of self-harm and determining appropriate responses. Taking note of self-harming behaviours is undoubtedly important when looking at the prevention of violence against the self or suicide as it provides the opportunity for intervention and support.

Diekstra's (1987) explanation of motivational factors has contributed to understandings of levels of violence against the self. He suggests that motives can be considered to be direct or indirect and that there is a clear relationship between motives and outcomes. Direct motives refer to a wish to end the conscious experience of the here-and-now situation with the expectation that death or cessation of consciousness will follow. Indirect motives refer to attempts to appeal to, or mobilize others to respond to the person's distress. Connections between direct and indirect motivation are captured by Schneidman (1987) and he refers to the embedded ambivalence of an individual cutting their own throat and crying for help at the same time and being genuine about both of these acts.

When only indirect motives are present, a key explanation can be maximizing the reaction of others. Talk or behaviour that is used as a last resort to influence others is frequently referred to as 'manipulative' or 'attention seeking'. When motives have been indirect or a combination of both indirect and direct and the reaction of others has been negative (dismissive, angry, punitive, blaming and guilt provoking), Diekstra (1987) observes that the individual may become even more determined to end their life by creating a shift in the balance between their indirect and direct motives. The increase in an individual's determination to cease consciousness on a permanent basis can directly flow from no longer believing they will succeed in mobilizing a positive response. The shift in motives from indirect, to both indirect and direct, to only direct motives can, as Diekstra (1987) points out, be associated with increased lethality.

However, it needs to be emphasized that excessive focus on determining 'whether they were or weren't really serious in their attempt' can ignore the levels of ambivalence operating and may lead to inappropriate and counterproductive responses from family and/or friends. Challenging the beliefs of others and the language they use to describe violence against the self is one simple avenue for change. If behaviour, categorized by some as 'attention seeking' or 'manipulative' is reframed as 'attention needing' it is more likely that empathic engagement will occur.

Violence against the self: the big picture

Suicide or violence against the self has taken place throughout history and across all countries. World Health Organization statistics indicate that there is one suicidal death every 40 seconds worldwide and that in the year 2000 approximately one million people died from suicide. This represents a global suicide rate of 16 per 100,000 (World Health Organization). There has been a 60 per cent increase in the rate of suicide worldwide in the past fifty years (Mohanty, Sahu, Mohanty and Patnaik, 2006), but the intersection of psychological, biological, social and environmental factors result in differing prevalence and behavioural features (for example, causes, timing, methods used) in different countries. The rates of reported suicide per 100,000 vary from 0 for both males and females (in Honduras, Antigua and Barbadu) to as high as 74.3 per 100,000 (for males in Lithuania) and 16.8 per 100,000 (for females in Sri Lanka). The following WHO suicide rates (per 100,000) provide a snapshot of trends worldwide (see Table 13.1).

These statistics provide a useful indicator, but it has to be borne in mind that the WHO figures are dependent on reports provided by individual countries and cannot necessarily be assumed to accurately reflect the real incidence of violence against the self worldwide. Very low rates may be the result of underreporting or misclassification, for example, as accidental deaths (Lester and Yang, 2005). Explanations for particularly high rates are not easily provided. Although it may

Table 13.1 Suicide rates (per 100,000 of population)

Country	Year	Male	Female
Australia	2001	20.1	5.3
Canada	2001	18.7	5.2
China (Hong Kong SAR)	2002	20.7	10.2
Finland	2003	31.9	9.8
France	2001	26.6	9.1
Israel	2000	9.9	2.7
Ireland	2001	21.4	4.1
Japan	2002	35.2	12.8
Norway	2002	16.1	5.8
Russian Federation	2002	69.3	11.9
Switzerland	2001	26.5	10.6
United Kingdom	2002	10.8	3.1
United States	2001	17.6	4.1

Source: World Health Organization, 2006a

be tempting to offer political explanations for the extremely high male Lithuanian rates, due to Lithuania's complex political history, this is not possible due to the lack of identifiable trends during the various political upheavals and the likelihood that multiple causative factors are at play.

A plausible culturally based contributing factor is the social attitude to suicide or violence against the self displayed in particular contexts at particular points in time. It is also notable that although governmental responses may vary, specific policies and campaigns can have an impact. An example is the way in which the World Suicide Prevention Day (an initiative of the International Association for Suicide Prevention and co-sponsored by WHO) resulted in numerous projects, campaigns and activities aimed at raising awareness about violence against the self in a range of countries.[1]

A number of population groups which include indigenous communities, immigrant and refugee groupings and ethnic communities, statistically appear to be at greater risk of violence against the self or suicide as a result of major power imbalances resulting from a history of colonialism and marginalization. Suicide among native populations is a significant issue worldwide and affects Native Americans, Canadian Inuit, Alaskan Natives, Aboriginal Australians and Native Hawaiians (Tester and McNicoll, 2004).

Youth suicide has also been highlighted as a key area of concern. In Australia, government policy and funding has started to take note of this area and the National Youth Suicide Prevention Strategy (NYSPS), implemented during 1995–9,

1 Notably in Australia, Austria, Belgium, Brazil, Canada, Chile, Germany, Ghana, Guam, Hong Kong, India, Ireland, Italy, Japan, Mexico, Nepal, Netherlands, New Zealand, Norfolk Island, Norway, Pakistan, Switzerland, Taiwan, Tanzania, Turkey, United Kingdom and Uruguay.

has been linked with a reduction in the violence against self or suicide rates of young Australian males in the 20–34 year age group. Since 1997–8, the number of incidents has declined from approximately 40 per 100,000 to approximately 20 per 100,000 in 2003 (Morrell, Page and Taylor, 2006). Current Australian initiatives are focusing more broadly on male suicide, in recognition that 80 per cent of all suicides are males, and 50 per cent of these are males aged 25–44 years. The National Forum on Men and Suicide, held in May 2006, produced a blueprint for a National Positive Health and Well Being Strategy, with the aim of assisting men to value themselves and their contribution to society, providing access to services, and challenging structural and policy barriers that prevent or inhibit such access (Suicide Prevention Australia, 2006).

Developing policy around such complex issues as preventing violence against the self is not easy and may be met with considerable resistance when it impinges on daily lives of many community members – for example gun control in Canada (Leenaars, De Leo, Goldney, Gulbinat and Wallace, 1998). Policies may also not have the impact intended. The passage of the Criminal Code Amendment (Suicide Related Material Offences) Act 2005 in the Australian Parliament, that came into force on 6 January 2006, can be taken as a pertinent example here. This legislation makes it a criminal offence to provide certain information about suicide. The intention of the Act is to limit the availability of information that might assist anyone in a suicide attempt. It prohibits 'possessing, controlling, producing, supplying or obtaining suicide related material [which] … directly or indirectly … counsels or incites committing or attempting to commit suicide' ('Criminal Code Amendment (Suicide Related Material Offences) Act 2005', 2006). This Act would appear to offer an effective means of shutting down websites such as those operating in Japan that promote group suicide pacts and include detailed descriptions of effective suicide methods (Hitosugi, Nagai and Tokudome, 2007). However, an unexpected consequence has been the closure of at least one very extensive suicide resource website. Its creators are concerned about the vague wording of the act, and the threat of considerable financial penalties (up to AUD$110,000 for each offence) if the website content was seen to be in breach of the Act. This voluntary closure may well be an over-reaction, but it can be used to demonstrate how a measure designed to address a specific problem, can by default, create others.

Policy and practice issues can be seen to be compounded when working with people from culturally and linguistically diverse backgrounds. Using western models of risk assessment and management often excludes rather than include. Women and men from culturally and linguistically diverse groups are often reluctant to work with interpreters. This is the case particularly when their circumstances involve interpersonal violence, which has been shown to be frequently associated with violence against the self (Stewart, 2006). This increases the 'possibility of misinterpreting suicidal signs and/or trauma because of a lack of familiarity with a client's cultural context [despite] … a genuine willingness … to guard against ethnocentrism in service delivery' (Stewart, 2006: 12–13). As has been seen in other chapters, the fear and shame associated with disclosing experiences of trauma and violence from within marginalized groups together with a distrust of statutory services, frequently prevents many from utilizing mental health services. Stewart (2006) suggests that services provided by non-government organizations are more likely to be accessed due to their greater flexibility, more appropriate service delivery approaches, and the increased likelihood that trust has been developed towards community-based organizations (Stewart, 2006).

The reluctance to seek help is not restricted to people of culturally and linguistically diverse backgrounds. It has been estimated that within the general population, 90 per cent of people who take their own life have a diagnosable mental disorder (NSW Department of Health, 2004). However, relatively few seek out professional mental health services, and even though they may have seen a general practitioner prior to a suicide attempt. As discussed in Chapter 2, 'Women and violence', this may be related to a distrust of statutory services and a fear of losing control over events.

When considering the frequency of violence against the self in the general community, it is clear that the responses of family and friends have the potential to significantly influence outcomes. In this, it is notable that research shows that a previous suicide attempt has been found to be a powerful predictor of further attempts with the likelihood of further attempts being associated with the reactions of family and friends (Farberow, 1994; Maris, 1991). As Appleby (1995) points out cries for help can be manifested in various ways and it is important for significant others to recognize the seriousness of the situation and to respond. A further point to note it that research has indicated that those clinically diagnosed as suffering from 'depression' are more likely to commit a violent act against the self during the period when they are starting to recover than at other times (Shneidman and Mandelkorn, 1994).

Dramatically detailed and frequent or extended media coverage of suicide, particularly of well-known media celebrities, has sometimes led to an apparent increase in incidents of violence against the self. Analysis of census and coroner's suicide data in Hong Kong, revealed an apparent increase in deaths due to suicide, particularly within a subgroup of males aged 25–39 years, following the extensive reporting of the suicide of a famous male pop singer in 2003. Connections between the suicides and the celebrity who'd suicided, were made as a result of the mention of the celebrity in some suicide notes, and the apparent copying of the method of suicide (Yip, Fu, Yang, *et al.*, 2006). Likewise in Quebec, there was an apparent increase in suicide after the detailed media coverage of the suicide of a well-known reporter (Tousignant, Mishara, Caillaud, Fortin and St-Laurent, 2005). However, the suicide of Kurt Cobain, the lead singer in the well-known band called Nirvana, was not similarly influential on suicide rates, with no evidence in either the United States or Australia, to suggest an increase in the rate of suicide. The reason for these differences is thought to be due to either the way in which the death was reported or 'the way the death was handled by Courtney Love, Cobain's widow and mother to his child, [which] may have assisted a negative response to the suicide' (Martin, 1998: 58).

It would be reckless to suggest that there is no connection between celebrity violence against the self, media coverage and an increase in suicide activity, but also presumptive to suggest that the connection is a straightforward causal one. Inappropriate media coverage is most likely to be a precipitating contributory factor. For some individuals the appeal of a potentially 'romantic' identification with a celebrity is an opportunity to create a meaningful connection, albeit in death, with another significant person. This motivation may therefore hasten the shift from ambivalence regarding violence against the self, to direct motives leading to a lethal attempt.

Martin (1998) comments that the features of media reporting most frequently associated with violence against the self include those instances where details are provided in various media forms and where the reports are repeated or explicit. He also comments that incidents which make the front page and which appear to glorify the self-directed violence and describe the method, are particularly influential.

To counteract such adverse effects, various suicide prevention organizations have developed media guidelines that have been accepted at a national level (for example, Canada, Japan). Martin (1998) suggests that it may be more productive to work with the media on providing information on constructive as opposed to tragic outcomes and to also ensure that all media reports include contact details for support organizations.

A further consideration is the effect that violence against the self can have on family or community groups. There can be seen to be a close parallel between potential consequences following 'sensational' media coverage and potential consequences following elaborate memorial services, particularly when it involves the suicide of a young person. The intention of memorials is generally to honour the deceased, and provide public expression of grief and regret for the loss of a loved one. However, the message when attending such a service, for someone who is feeling powerless, disregarded and unimportant and who may already have considered acts of self-violence is that in death, they too may be equally honoured and publicly lauded and respected.

Implications for human service professionals

It is important for human service providers to focus on preventative strategies and also to be able to put support systems in place when warning signs are noted. The actual crisis of an imminent suicide attempt is often short-lived and may be averted through vigilance, by seeking professional help and the removal of weapons or the means by which the person had planned their violent act against the self. Supportive strategies need also to be directed towards creating a change in the factors or circumstances that contributed to desire to inflict violence upon the self. This may require professional help and the extended intervention of friends and family. In relation to the latter group, it is essential to garner the involvement of appropriate others to share the emotional load of supporting an individual in crisis, being available and accessible for as long as is necessary, can be very stressful for any one person.

As has been seen, the statistics relating to violence against the self vary from country to country. More recently, attention has turned to determining the protective factors that enhance coping and resilience as a means of suicide prevention. Good self-esteem, having a sense of belonging and an articulated belief system are protective factors associated with resilience and coping. Assisting people, particularly young people to respect themselves, by offering social support and connection, acceptance and appreciation, opportunities to achieve in areas which they and others value and to develop problem-solving skills, can lead to sustainable feelings of worth and acceptance. These are the basis of resilience and coping. When combined with a sense of meaning and purpose, resilience creates the optimistic reality that 'He who has a *why* to live for, can bear with almost any *how*' (Nietzsche cited in Frankl, 1963: xi).

Chapter summary

Violence against the self: self-harm and suicide

- Violence against the self has a worldwide relevance.
- Experiences of oppression, disempowerment, disconnectedness, physical and psychological abuse, are frequently linked with violence against the self.
- No one theory is able to account for violence against the self.
- The causes of violence against the self are complex, but many instances are preventable.
- Policies worldwide are mixed, but there is evidence to show that targeted activity has a positive outcome.
- Good self-esteem, having a sense of belonging and an articulated belief system are protective factors associated with resilience and coping.

14 Disability and violence

Barbara Fawcett

Historically, connections have been made between appearance, even minor impairments and violence. Macaulay said of Titus Oates,

> his short neck, his legs uneven … as those of a badger, his forehead low as that of a baboon, his purple cheeks, and his monstrous length of chin … those hideous features on which villainy seemed to be written by the hand of God.
>
> (Macaulay's History of England 1855–61, 1906 edition)

This quote draws attention to how physical impairment has been negatively viewed throughout the ages whilst at the same time also being seen as an indicator of 'villainy' or various forms of violence. This chapter will begin by providing an historical overview of how disability has been both understood and responded to. Conceptualizations of disability will then be explored and the links and association which can be made between these and issues concerning oppression, abuse and violence will be examined. Although the discussion can be seen to primarily relate to western countries, there are direct associations which can be made with non-western countries although greater emphasis has of necessity to be placed on significant resource differentials. It also has to be borne in mind that matters raised in other chapters relate to disabled women and men in the same way as they do to other individuals and social groupings.

Historical overview

With regard to conceptualizations of disability, as highlighted in the quote by Macaulay, throughout the ages connections have been made between 'disability' and devalued characteristics. In Ancient Sparta for example, babies who did not satisfy the stringent demands of the Gerousia were left to die on mountainsides. Christian doctrine has variously regarded 'disability' as a cross to bear, as a punishment for past sins, as a sign of tainted blood, or occasionally as a gift from God to be cherished and cared for. The Enlightenment period championed the cause of science, logic, rationality and progress. Physical impairment gradually became the preserve of medicine and attention was directed towards defining and categorizing specific conditions. Individuals were seen to be disabled by their impairment and responses incorporated diagnostic examination, classification, treatment, 'care' and increasingly, segregation. This was influenced by and in turn influenced the capacity of the increasingly industrialized workforce to meet the needs of those less able to pull their weight financially. These factors promoted the growth of large-scale institutions where over time, particularly given the influence of the Eugenics movement, the purpose was related as much to protecting the general public from 'abnormal contaminating elements as it was about caring for those requiring personal assistance.

Large-scale residential establishments continued to dominate provision for disabled women and men until the 1960s when the work of Goffman (1961), and Robb (1967), amongst others drew attention to how institutions routinely fostered abusive acts and practices. Reports condemning the ill-treatment of 'patients' in institutions such as South Ockendon Hospital (HMSO, 1974) in the United Kingdom and Callan Park Hospital (McClemens Report, 1961) in NSW, Australia, together with the increasing costs of institutional facilities and pharmaceutical advances which made segregation less justifiable, resulted in pressure for change. Emphasis gradually came to be placed on 'care in the community' as a means of countering the effects of institutionalized practices and promoting an 'ordinary life' for disabled people. However, 'community care' has come to mean very different things for different individuals. For some, it has evolved into independent living schemes, controlled and operated by disabled people. Many of these, such as the Derbyshire scheme in the UK (Davis, 1993), were based on Centre for Independent Living Services which were developed in the United States. These promoted the direct involvement of disabled people in community based services, challenged stereotypes and campaigned for citizenship rights. For others, it has resulted in struggles to obtain the personal and financial assistance required. It has also become clear that in some instances, for those who moved into residential care settings in the community, old institutional practices continued on a smaller scale. Biggs, Phillipson and Kingston (1995), for example, have demonstrated connections between 'institutions' and institutional practices within residential settings in the community. In particular they have drawn attention to how the use of functional assessments linked to rating scales, residents being given limited opportunity for self-determination and independent socialization, and the operation of rigid routines, can reproduce passivity and dependency and foster a climate of control. Peace, Kellaher and Willcocks (1997) have pointed to the positive changes which have taken place in residential settings over the last decade in countries such as the United Kingdom, but have also highlighted how easily enabling environments can regress into disabling regimes. Disability rights movements and the social model of disability were borne out of frustration and dissatisfaction with residential 'care' practices which even at their best were seen as condemning disabled people to a lifetime of care, control and dependency. These practices were regarded as privileging individual and medical responses to impairment and as prioritizing pathologizing forms of intervention (Finkelstein, 1991).

Dissatisfaction with such responses has resulted in proponents of disability rights movements pertinently stating that residential care workers and social and health care professionals have to be regarded as part of the problem unless they fully engage with service users in promoting self-autonomy and self-determination (Oliver and Sapey, 2006).

Conceptualizations of disability

Since the 1980s definitions, understandings and assumptions about 'disability' and about the linkages between disability, violence and abuse have changed radically. The emergence of a social model of disability with sociological underpinnings has served to bring into sharp relief and also challenge understandings which categorized disabled women and men on the basis of their individual impairment and which limited expectations to either continually striving for independence or to receiving 'care'. Social model orientations highlight how disabled people are disabled, not by individual impairments, but at all levels by oppressive social, economic, political and cultural practices. Emphasis has been placed on the importance of individual autonomy, which is about disabled people being in control of what happens to them without necessarily doing everything themselves. There is also a focus on a rights-based approach to citizenship entitlements to publicly display disparities between disabled and non-disabled people and to campaign for resources and equality.

Social model understandings of disability have resulted in marked changes in conceptualizations of disability in western countries particularly and have promoted the enactment of disability rights legislation and changes in service provision. Even where service provision in countries appears resistant to change, social model understandings have provided a viable alternative model that can be used to mount effective challenges to practices regarded by consumers as unhelpful. However, the social model of disability is not a static entity and is also subject to challenge and change. An example is that during the 1980s and the early 1990s presentations of the social model of disability focused on portraying 'disability' as a homogeneous entity with a unified constituency and a singular message. This assumption that the social model represented all disabled people was countered by Dalley (1993) who drew attention to the previously unacknowledged influence of younger, impaired, but fit white men. Since that time, universalist claims have been modified and matters of difference and diversity with regard to personal experience, gender issues and ethnicity have been acknowledged. The political message of the social model presented by disability rights movements remains clear and unambiguous, but at conceptual levels discussion has become more nuanced and theoretically engaging.

However, there are two areas in particular which remain contentious and these have a bearing on discussions about disability and oppression. These relate to the ways in which 'oppression' has been conceptualized and the place of experience within this conceptualization.

The social model of disability makes a direct association between disability and oppression and as highlighted, the social model with its emphasis on social, political, civil and cultural rights is used a means of drawing attention to discrepancies and to the extent of the discrimination experienced. However, it is notable that the early tendency to list oppressions in order to emphasize the specific positions occupied has retained currency. Accordingly, the phrase 'double oppression' coined by Begum, Hill and Stevens in 1994 is still used to refer to being black and disabled. Similarly, the term 'triple oppression' put forward by Begum in 1992 to refer to being female, black and disabled continues to be applied. However, as Fawcett (2000)[1] has pointed out these listings can be double-edged. They can serve as a useful point of reference for the individual concerned, or can be regarded as a means of stereotypically categorizing an individual on the basis of taken-for-granted assumptions. They can also be regarded as promoting a victim-orientated emphasis and, at individual and social levels, as projecting a negative and passive identity.

It is notable that the prioritizing of personal experiences has been associated with the 'second wave' feminist slogan, 'the personal is political', to emphasize gender differences and to bring personal experiences within disability rights movements into the campaign for citizenship rights for disabled people. However, this has provoked controversy with regard to whether an individual has to have an impairment(s) and experience of disabilism in order to maintain an effective challenge. It has also promoted a form of competitiveness in relation to whose experience can be seen to be the most valid. The privileging of personal experience is clearly related to concerns about the appropriation of the political message if non-disabled others have a significant voice. However, the dangers of marginalization and further exploitation remain ever present in this approach (Fawcett, 2000).

This discussion promotes an examination of the associations which can be made between oppression, violence and abuse. The social model of disability rejects arguments which make connections between disability and increased vulnerability. Such associations are regarded as linking characteristics such as high physical assistance needs and frailty with violent or abusive responses and as privileging pathologizing explanations. However, the message put forward by disability rights movements that disabled individuals are disabled not by impairments but by individual and organizational prejudice and discrimination, also begs the question about whether disabled women and men are more likely to be subject to violence and abuse because of the pervasive oppressive forces operating. In attempting to formulate a response to this question, it is possible to assert that for disabled women and men rather than there being a clear distinction which can be made between oppression, abuse and violence, there is a blurring into what can be described as a revolving circle. Routinized practices, associated with patterns of care in domestic and residential settings, can so easily become restrictive, controlling and rigid. Violent and abusive acts can slide into becoming routine and can be justified in the name of compliance. Morris (1996) has emphasized the importance of reciprocal

---

1 Fawcett in *Feminist Perspectives on Disability* (2000), has critically explored similarities between 'second wave feminisms' and disability rights movements.

caring relationships where 'care' is defined in the broad sense of 'caring about' and where trust, sharing and strengths, not weaknesses, are emphasized. 'Caring' relationships, perceived and operated as unidimensional, rather than multidimensional, where responsibility for physical assistance falls unilaterally on the shoulders of a family member or a small group of poorly paid and overstretched care workers and where there are overt or covert power imbalances operating, clearly contain within them the potential for a variety of oppressive, abusive and violent acts. However, the provision of training, support, resources and personal assistance and direct payments for services being controlled by the disabled person, whatever the setting, can prevent the unacceptable being rendered acceptable and pre-empt the crossing of boundaries from 'care' into abuse. Abusive practices can be fostered by institutional constraints and can be perpetuated by systems where disabled people are not in control of their personal support needs.

A further related question that can be posed and which corresponds to the underpinning point behind Begum's argument (1992), is concerned with whether disabled women are more likely to be subject to violence and abuse than disabled men. It is notable that a study carried out by Kvam and Braathen (2006) which focused on the violence and abuse of disabled women in Malawi, used as its starting point the assumption that disabled women are more likely to be subject to violations of their human rights than non-disabled women. The study was based on the premise that much abuse is hidden and that there is a lot of stigma and shame connected with disability. Its purpose was to improve the living conditions of disabled women in Malawi by disclosing and describing the nature and extent of the abuse, neglect, violence and discrimination experienced. The results of the study, given that it had a qualitative orientation, cannot be seen to be representative, but the findings were not those expected. The study did not find evidence of physical or sexual ill-treatment or abuse of disabled girls within families, although several of the participants disclosed that they had been sexually exploited by a non-family member. Rather than individual instances of violence and abuse coming to the fore, the participants drew attention to how the extra costs of disability exacerbated family poverty and how existing health provision did not cater for disabled women. They also drew attention to how they were excluded from education and from valued forms of social life and how they, as disabled women, had no public presence and were largely rendered invisible.

This study highlights how expectations and findings can differ substantially. To further explore the question of whether disabled women are more likely to be subject to violent and abusive acts than disabled men, it is also useful to look at the various ways in which disabled women can be portrayed. These different perspectives could be viewed as occupying positions on a continuum. At one end disabled women could be regarded as a diverse, yet vulnerable group requiring associated programmes of assessment and intervention to protect them from intimate partner violence in a home environment or from a variety of forms of individual and systemic abuse in a residential establishment. At the other end of the continuum, disabled women could be portrayed as being subject to ongoing social political, cultural and political abuse as a result of disabling/oppressive barriers of prejudice, discrimination and oppression. There could clearly also be a range of positions in between. An exploration of these perspectives brings to the fore a number of pertinent considerations.

It has been highlighted in Chapter 2, 'Women and violence', that gendered power imbalances can make the possibility of intimate partner violence more likely, but not inevitable in some contexts but not in others. Relationships, where aspects of dependency (whether financial or linked to forms of physical assistance) are emphasized or given structural reinforcement, will have an increased tendency to result in strengthening rather than countering gendered power imbalances and increasing the possibility of psychological control, physical violence and various forms of routinized abuse. However, if it is accepted that in some sets of circumstances disabled women are more susceptible to violence and abuse than disabled men or non-disabled women, then the next question to pose is what would constitute an appropriate response? To look at an hypothetical scenario, if a disabled women, living in her own home or in a residential setting discloses that she has been subject to violence and/or abuse and requests assistance, then the matter appears fairly clear cut, although 'assistance' which results in the woman losing control over what subsequently happens to her, could easily transform what the woman would regard as supportive assistance into a form of oppressive management. The ways in which forms of intervention can so easily slide into becoming an additional oppressive barrier rather than providing constructive support also becomes apparent if another version of this scenario is presented. If, for example, a worker, friend or professional identifies a disabled woman as being vulnerable to violence or abuse and takes action without the full involvement and agreement of the woman concerned, then again this intervention could be construed as restrictive and controlling. Mullender and Hague (2001) have drawn attention to the importance of support systems, the availability of help lines, and the provision of accessible information which both names and condemns violence and abuse. They also emphasize how women survivors of violence and abuse want services where they are actively consulted about their needs, where they receive support in taking the action which they regard as appropriate and where women survivors of abuse are employed by support agencies and service providers.

Looking at the other end of the continuum and emphasizing the political message contained in the social model of disability, disabled women can be seen to be discriminated against both socially and materially. Middleton (1999) makes the point that all aspects of discrimination can be regarded as evidence of abuse. This can relate to disabled women being regarded as incapable of being 'good' mothers, to disabled women not being able to live their lives in the way they would want because of limited or restrictive services, to disabled women having to contend with increasing family pressure as a result of having to rely on family members to provide daily physical assistance. Abuse can also feature in accepted medical practices. Westcott (1998) has explored how disabled girls in particular are not asked to give permission for medical examinations and how difficult it is for a disabled girl to refuse a medical intervention. She highlights how such routinized 'handling' can translate into a disabled girl or woman believing that they cannot say no. This in turn, easily slides into the perpetration of intentional sexual abuse. This discussion draws attention to how disabled women, viewed as a heterogeneous group, are more likely to be subject to forms of violence and abuse than disabled men.

However, it does also need to be pointed out, that women too can become perpetrators of abuse in both domestic and residential settings. This abuse can be routinized and sanctioned by local justifications. The numbers comparatively are small and arguments about male victims have often been used as a means of resisting positive action for women. Nevertheless, in all settings situational factors combined with stereotypical prejudices and assumptions, limited access to education, training and support mechanisms and a lack of economic and social resources, can all play a part. The interaction of these factors can produce ablebodied/non-ablebodied power and resource differentials which can so easily operate to negative effect.

Implications for human service professionals

The involvement of human service professionals in the identification of vulnerability can bring to the fore particularly problematic and difficult aspects for disabled women and men. It can, on the one hand, be viewed as an important means of obtaining external protection, on the other it can be regarded as undermining the rights and the self-determination of the individual. As highlighted, proponents of the social model of disability have stressed that terms such as 'dependence', 'independence' and 'vulnerability' are a legacy of medicalized or individualized understandings of disability and as such are constraining and oppressive. However, notwithstanding this, most western nations have developed or are developing multi-agency procedures and staff training strategies to address the abuse of 'vulnerable' adults. These positions can appear to be polarized, although as depicted in the hypothetical scenario given above, it is the associated action with regard to who directs events, which has to be seen as the most important consideration. Oliver and Sapey (2006) make it clear that professional activity should be directed towards tackling disabling factors such as poverty, poor housing, employment issues and unhelpful social responses rather than the management of an impairment. They also emphasize the importance of maintaining a strong link between theory and practice. A focus on individualized, clinical approaches will clearly direct intervention down a certain path, whilst connections made with what Oliver and Sapey (2006) term 'the social problem theory of disability', directs activity towards social action. Such action views professionals as facilitators and 'determined advocates' ensuring, for example, that personal assistants are available to work under the direction of the disabled person. Emphasis is also placed on disabled people operating as their own keyworkers and on direct payment schemes and independent living schemes being further promoted as a means of reinforcing autonomy and self-direction.

In conclusion, it is important to emphasize that many within disability movements have argued for professionals to adopt a community, not a clinical focus and to work in real partnership with disabled people promoting equality, citizenship entitlements and social justice. This is a challenge for professionals and one which their training might not have equipped them for. However, in relation to overcoming oppression, abuse and violence towards disabled people this constitutes a clear and unambiguous way forward and one which positively counters institutional and individual entrenched positions and attitudes.

Chapter summary

Disability and violence

- Historically, disabled people have been subject to wide-ranging abuse, oppression and violence.
- Largely, but not exclusively as a result of abusive acts and routinized oppressive practices coming to light in the 1960s, 'community care' or 'care in the community' gained currency.
- Social model orientations have promoted citizenship rights, autonomy and self-determination and have challenged oppressive policies and practices.
- The use of experience within the social model to draw attention to the extent of the oppression can be seen to be double-edged. On the one hand it can serve as a useful point of reference. On the other, it can promote a victim-orientated emphasis and a passive identity.
- Links between disability and increased vulnerability can promote pathological explanations.
- Disabled women and men are more likely to be subject to violence and abuse as a result of individual prejudice and discrimination.
- Personal assistance, if not under the direct control of the disabled person can easily slide, whatever the setting, into restrictive, controlling and rigid practices and oppressive management.
- At an international level, disabled women can be seen to be subject to more oppressive barriers and to be more susceptible to violent acts than disabled men.
- With regard to human service professionals, emphasis is placed on the importance of social issues, on advocacy, on autonomy and self-direction, and upon professionals operating in this area adopting a community as opposed to a clinical focus.

15 Older people and violence

Lindsey Napier and Fran Waugh

The purpose of this chapter is to provide an overview of violence against older people, a field that has been the subject of systematic professional enquiry for over thirty years. First, we provide a brief overview of the social position of older people in the twenty-first century. Second, a summary of the emergence of abuse of older people as an acknowledged social problem is outlined. Third, we concentrate on identifying four ways in which older people have been or are characterized with respect to their experience of violence, abuse and oppression, namely as victims of abuse, as persons subject to criminal acts, as vulnerable persons and as rights bearing citizens. We then elaborate how these different conceptualizations lead to different human service responses before turning to the emerging voices of older people themselves. We end by arguing for local approaches to be rights-based, responsive to political, economic and cultural contexts.

Older people in the twenty-first century

In this paper we adopt the World Health Organization's definition of older people as persons 60 years and over (WHO and The International Network for the Prevention of Elder Abuse [INPEA], 2002). Due to the dramatic improvements in healthcare, work conditions, general standards of living and a drop in fertility rates across most societies, the world's population is ageing (Department of Economic and Social Affairs, United Nations, 2004). In general, the 'demographic transition' to ageing societies as a worldwide trend poses many challenges for governments, families and communities throughout the world, one of these being violence against older people.

The proportion of people aged 60 years and over is increasing: 'Predictions indicated that by 2025 the global population of [persons 60 years and over] will double to 1.2 billion' (WHO and INPEA, 2002: 2). Every month one million people turn 60 with 80 per cent of these in the developing countries. The demographic profile is country specific. The trend takes several forms affected by the relative stability or collapse of birth rates, rising or falling death rates, rates of immigration and the inter-relation of all these. Australia for example is ageing relatively slowly, neither as extensively as older European states, nor as rapidly as parts of Asia. In China, for example, the proportion of people aged 60 years is estimated to double to 200 million between 2005 and 2015 and by 2050 a third of the population in China is expected to be retired (French, 2007). In South Korea the aged population doubled from 1.45 million in 1980 to 3 million in 2000 (Kyeung and Warnes, 2001). In contrast France took 115 years to double its aged population, the United Kingdom 70 years and Japan over 30 years (Kyeung and Warnes, 2001). However, in Australia there has been an 114 per cent increase over the past two decades of people aged 85 years and over from 1 per cent to 1.5 per cent in 2004 (Phillips and Kendig, forthcoming).

Women are the majority of the older population in virtually all nations. Globally men continue to die several years before women. Worldwide in 2000–5, women's life expectancy was 68 years, five years more than men (Department of Economic and Social Affairs, United Nations, 2004). This gap was larger in developed countries, seven years compared with two years in least developed countries. The exception to this is in Southern Africa (such as Botswana, Lesotho and Swaziland) where the impact of HIV/AIDS, has resulted in a decline in life expectancy from 62 years in 1990–5 to 48 years in 2000–5 (Department of Economic and Social Affairs, United Nations, 2004).

Inequalities in both developing and developed societies persist into older age and may be deepening. In Australia, for example, a person of Aboriginal, Torres Strait Islander descent dies on an average 20 years before their Australian counterpart (Phillips and Kendig, forthcoming). Social inequalities and injustices continue into older age. For instance, if older women have not been able to own their accommodation, save money in preparation for their older age, because of a lack of education, lack of employment opportunities, unpaid caregiving roles, discrimination or a history of violence, then their poverty is often compounded in older age (Phillips, 2006). End-of-life does not suddenly provide a level playing field. Thirty per cent of the world's aged are not in receipt of pension schemes (WHO and INPEA, 2002).

The social world of older people is a rapidly changing one, in both developing and developing societies. Factors which have contributed to this include increased participation of women in the paid employment, urbanization and a widening of the gap between the rich and the poor (WHO and INPEA, 2002). The opening up of free trade and the rise of successful economies has not universally benefited older people. For instance, the aspirations of a rising urban middle class in India have led to rising living standards, rising pressures to establish own households, rising expectations for young women to lead lives outside the domestic sphere and increasing disintegration of multigenerational households. Pressure on older people to sacrifice their family home is reported as a primary cause of violence (Page, 2006).

Old people may encompass both positive and negative value positions. In developed and developing countries positive values are placed on the family as ideally caring for its dependent members who are considered to be valued members of society. In contrast, negative values are expressed through ageism when older people are viewed as unproductive and dependent and are seen as different from the rest of society. They are labelled as 'the problem' especially if they are poor and excluded as social citizens. This may be compounded by sexism, heterosexism and racism. These negative values combined with the before mentioned social changes contribute to a climate where violence against older people is cultivated.

Attention to violence

Violence against older people in the family home was first described as 'granny battering' in the 1970s. Attention to such violence emerged simultaneously alongside forms of family violence, particularly violence towards children and women. In the United Kingdom Biggs (1995), has claimed that violence towards older people did not receive the priority accorded to children and women, whom he claimed were perceived to be at the centre rather than the margins of society. However, at this time a House Select Committee on Ageing enquiry in the United States put 'elder abuse' firmly within the mandate of adult protective services (O'Connor and Rowe, 2005). This led to a burgeoning official interest in identifying the incidence and the prevalence and by 1982 elder abuse had been raised to international level of concern in the United Nations Principles for Older Persons (Resolution 37/51) where, it was asserted: 'seniors have a right to live free from neglect, exploitation or abuse'.

The term elder abuse appears to have emerged as a favoured term for two reasons. It both fitted an existing stereotype of the older person as marginal and it described a multidimensional and multi-causal experience. Official preoccupation with defining its nature and prevalence and determining concomitant official responses followed. By the end of the 1980s, when countries like Australia and Sweden were also paying attention to the phenomenon, the response was professionally driven. The debate focused on whether or not to introduce mandatory reporting, whether to prioritize institutional abuse in the light of the move to community care, what relation if any existed between domestic violence and 'elder abuse'. The exposure of ageism and age discrimination had also commenced.

Kinnear and Graycar (1999) note that there are ongoing debates in Australia about defining elder abuse as there is minimal consensus as how to define harm. For example, they provide the definition of elder abuse as, 'any behaviour or pattern of behaviours by a person or persons which results in harm to an older person' (Kinnear and Graycar,1999: 2). Australian studies have tended to include categories such as physical abuse; emotional or psychological abuse; neglect, economic abuse, sexual abuse (Kinnear and Graycar, 1999). Self-neglect was omitted from definitions in Australia as all States and Territories in Australia could employ guardianship legislation to protect the older person who had diminished decision-making capacities due to dementia, for instance (Kinnear and Graycar, 1999).

Because of the debates in defining elder abuse the prevalence of elder abuse has been difficult to estimate. Kurrle (2004) notes that studies in Australia and overseas suggest between 4 to 10 per cent of patients referred to aged care services are victims of abuse. The World Health Organization and the International Network for the Prevention of Elder Abuse (2002) review of literature found that the prevalence for all types of abuse ranged from between 4 and 6 per cent (WHO and INPEA, 2002).

Different ways of understanding and responding to violence against older people

Following Harbison and Morrow (1998), we differentiate between older people being perceived as victims of abuse and being perceived as persons subject to illegal acts. We examine the consequences for older people now being termed 'vulnerable' by governments in the United Kingdom and in New South Wales before turning to the focus now being placed on elder abuse in developing as well as developed societies and the call for its being named as a basic human rights issue, including by older people themselves. For each of these concepts we consider the following questions: What explanation is being provided?; Who is providing the explanation; What is the strength of the evidence?; What is the impact on official policies and programmes?; and, What is the current status of the conceptualization?

Older people as victims of abuse

Consistent with theorizing of older age as a time of withdrawal and dependency, early attention to what came to be called elder abuse in the United States was underpinned by the assumption that older age ushers in dependency and impairment – functional impairments, physical, mental or both (Tomita, 2006). Sickness, frailty and decay left older people vulnerable – victim to the natural decline of old age. From the mid-1980s it was the psychopathology and dependency of abusers, for instance because of mental illness or drug and substance abuse, that claimed stronger explanatory power. Older people fell victim to abuse of family members who were dependent on them for money, accommodation, care, security. Carer stress subsequently provided a further explanation as to why an older person could be victim to abuse. As responsibility for caring was returned firmly to the informal sphere, to 'community' and 'family', and the demands placed on the emerging category of 'carers' better understood by professionals and articulated by carers themselves, the situational demands and frustrations associated with caring became a ready explanation for abuse. Such an explanation diverts attention from the older person, leads to primary identification with the perceived carer, especially when the victim may be perceived as 'burden'. Biggs has argued that carer stress became 'the most common folk explanation of elder mistreatment' (1993: 67). He has suggested that regardless of the emerging research evidence failing to support stress as a primary explanation, identification with the carer and the caring situation was easier for younger professionals and policy makers, given the low status accorded work with older people.

Rather than identifying older people as the victim, others have argued, as has Kurrle (2004) in Australia, that rather than tending to place the parties and their different needs in conflict, against each other, 'in many cases it may be more appropriate to look at the situation as one in which there are two victims, rather than a victim and an abuser' (Kurrle, 2004: 40). In combination with provision of community services, a counselling approach, with either or both parties, may achieve the older person becoming more capable of coping with and finding safety in their situation, without risking retaliation by the abuser (the other victim) or removal to residential care, often perceived as the only alternative.

Both victims are perceived to require professional management – detection, assessment and treatment. The focus is on care of both parties (Kinnear and Graycar, 1999) with attention placed on the interior of families, on interpersonal behaviours and often long-standing conflicts in domestic settings. There is an absence of an analysis of power and gender in this conceptualization.

Older people as subject to illegal acts

While it may be claimed that 'labeling harmful acts as "abuse" detracts from the criminality of the behaviour and degrades the experience of victims' (Kinnear and Graycar, 1999: 3), the 'discovery' of 'elder abuse' in the United States of America did lead to a legal requirement in most US states since 1988 to investigate suspected cases of elder abuse. This served to criminalize abuse, neglect and exploitation (Biggs, 1993). In countries like the United States and Australia, an older person suffering abuse commonly presents to the healthcare provider, however, where, arguably, the approach is one of determining needs and providing professional care, rather than a 'violence' approach and a pathway to the criminal justice system. Mandatory reporting may cut across this, requiring more than following protocols for multidisciplinary and interagency assessment and supportive interventions. Resorting to mandatory reporting is criticized for resting on the false assumption that there is one clear perpetrator and for potentially jeopardizing the self-determination of victims.

Nevertheless, moving from defining the problem as one of care, carers and the care relationship to one defining the actors as perpetrators and persons wronged by violent acts places the behaviour in a criminal justice framework. The abuse is redefined as a public act which is a crime, and moves it from the private domestic sphere. Being older is not of itself the primary issue. Neither is gender.

However, the one consistent finding is that the majority of older people who experience abuse are women. It is in belated recognition that older women also live and have lived with the experience and effects of domestic violence that dialogue has ensued between activists, providers and policy makers across the 'divide' of domestic violence and elder abuse. Penhale (2003) reports that it has only been in the last fifteen years that attention has been paid to the commonalities, differences and shared approaches to older women, domestic violence and elder abuse, with an accompanying call for greater understanding and cooperation between domestic violence and services for older women. The commonalities include the facts that: psychological and physical abuse go hand in hand: an older person is likely to internalize the denigration, to defend and protect the abuser, to maintain silence, and to be unable to imagine different circumstances.

Regardless of age, it is inappropriate to define these as problems of individual pathology. Rather, they must be understood as expressions of dominant social norms and attitudes: women as legitimately controlled by the social power of men and older people as legitimately regarded as redundant and dependent and whose social claims can therefore be ignored. What may differentiate older from younger women may include differing perceptions of what women can expect and be entitled to within marriage and 'the family'. Diminishing strength and resilience may also play a part in the will and capacity of older women to seek assistance to name and confront the abuse they experience as violence. An additional fear for an older person may be that being moved out of home into residential care will ensue, a fear that may well be realistic (McCreadie, 1996).

Collaboration between agencies is advocated as an important strategy to address these issues (Vinton, 2003). The construction of 'elder abuse' as violence, influenced by conversations with domestic violence, necessarily pushes policy makers to consider its criminalization.

Older people as vulnerable

In their introduction to the debate as to whether the safety and protection of older people can be enhanced through the criminalization of elder abuse, Kinnear and Graycar, assert that:

> Although research suggests that older people are less at risk of criminal victimization than other age groups, the incidents which do occur, as well as the fear of such events, can have a dramatic impact on the quality of life of those older people, especially those who are vulnerable due to physical frailty, dependency or social isolation. Of course not *all* older people are frail, dependent and vulnerable – the most remain independent and active community members for the latter years of their lives. Nevertheless, frailty, dependence and vulnerability do structure the lives and living patterns of a significant percentage of older people. (1999: 1)

We agree with this statement and note that the appeal to the term 'vulnerable' to describe many older people is not new. Current policy, notably in the United Kingdom and now under consideration in New South Wales (Roberson, personal communication) has adopted the term, in England to refer to persons in need of services. The document *No Secrets* (Department of Health, 2000) charged all English local authority social services departments to develop a multi-agency code of practice for the protection of vulnerable adults, and to work in partnership with other agencies to ensure consistent and effective responses. The Protection of Vulnerable Adults scheme for England and Wales followed, covering care homes and domiciliary agencies (Department of Health, 2004).

In New South Wales where the protocol refers to older people living 'in the community', that is outside residential care, several groups of older people are identified as being particularly vulnerable to risk of abuse, including women who have suffered domestic violence for many years. The defining characteristic is vulnerability. The aim of risk detection, protection and prevention can then be pursued in many ways, including through the criminal justice system. Channels of communication and accountability are exhaustively detailed in such documents. The emphasis is on targeted identification, investigation, assessment, monitoring and treatment of individuals, one of the risk paradigms identified by Taylor (2006).

The benefits of adopting a language of vulnerability may however be outweighed by unintended potential harm. For a start, while policy documents may use the term to refer to a particular group (those in need of services and unable to take care of themselves, for instance), there is a danger of older people as a group being characterized as vulnerable and once again passive – exposed to and passively subject to risks and threats, outside their control, albeit relatively more or less able to harness their coping capacity and withstand the threat. Of equal concern, perhaps, is that the structural dimensions of vulnerability may be overlooked: older people, just as others, are unequally 'prone to disaster' than others, reflecting broader inequalities, including gender inequalities. Again, defining older people as vulnerable and in need of professional protection risks overriding or ignoring their own priorities (Schröder-Butterfill and Marianti, 2006).

Older people as rights bearing citizens

Policy documents such as those above contend that adopting a language of vulnerability is consistent with a human rights approach to elder abuse. The draft revised New South Wales 'Interagency protocol for responding to abuse of older people' asserts that, 'Older people have the right to be treated with dignity and respect and to live in safe environment' (NSW Department of Ageing; Disability and Home Care Services 2007: 3). This is in keeping with the thrust of declarations of international forums, where elder abuse has increasingly been a focus of research and policy formulation. The Second World Assembly on Ageing in 2002 was an important milestone in the United Nations addressing the abuse of older persons in a global perspective (Commission for Social Development, UN; 2002a). At this meeting, the Commission for Social Development presented it with the proposition that abuse of older persons must be understood as a human rights issue.

The Commission proposed that rights could only be exercised when poverty eradication and reduction of violence were addressed in a complementary fashion. It noted that 'In many societies, older persons comprise a disproportionate number of the poor and of the poorest among the poor' (2002a: 3, 4). It asserted that it is imperative to address ageism and sexism – for the denigration and devaluing of older people to give way to equality of access to 'opportunities, resources and entitlements' (Commission for Social Development, UN, 2002a: 4). It widened the types of abuse to include community violence, political violence and armed conflict and HIV/AIDS-related violence, types particularly noted by Ferreira (2004) in her elaboration of the situation in Africa.

The Council argued that a framework for policy and action must be directly based on human rights. Such a framework would:

(a) draw attention to the political issues of abuse of older persons and discrimination
(b) challenge the abuse of economic and social means and entitlements of older persons
(c) consider effective responses to abuse and violence (Commission for Social Development, UN, 2002a: 3)

In a subsequent paper Ferreira (2004) explicated the situation in Africa, 'the world's poorest region', endorsing the views of Council and asserting that in Africa, the problem of elder abuse, to be understood as a human rights issue, is escalating. She drew attention to the situation – 'instability, wars and conflict; endemic corruption, weak leadership and poor management; calamities and disasters; and disease and epidemics' and to the dreadful position of older people, particularly widows. Here, she clarified, elder violence is increasingly the preferred term, reflecting its extreme nature – economic, community and political – with violence being perpetrated collectively, linked with a breakdown in social relations. For example, widows, who are most at risk and least able to resist, are being coerced into surrendering inheritance rights, in order to resolve conflict over property ownership. Much worse may befall a widow – she may be scapegoated as a witch, in order to explain mass disasters, and raped, ostracized and banished, on occasion tortured and even killed. The right asserted here is the claim to life.

Older people's voices

It can rightly be asked why we leave the voices of older people to the last part of this chapter. Why have policy makers and human service providers driven the agenda? Why, as the Secretary of the United Nations (Commision for Social Development, 2002a) has noted, are there so few studies documenting older people's perceptions and experiences of abuse?

In Canada, Harbison and Morrow (1998) had earlier highlighted the urgency of exploring such questions by pointing to the disabling consequences of early theorizing of older age as a time of disengagement and frailty and the state's positioning of older people as recipients rather than producers of services. They pointed out that pathologizing and medicalizing ageing had left little expectation that older people themselves would 'take up arms'. 'The ageing enterprise' (Estes, 1979) had much invested in constructing older people as essentially dependent. Governments now do exhort people approaching old age to remain healthy, self-reliant and contributory, of course; however, it may be no easier nowadays to speak about abuse and violence. As well, older people do not speak with one voice: different cohorts may have differing expectations of themselves, the family, marriage and the state. For the 'old old', the family may well be the sole institution looked to for assistance, and oneself, in silence, when the family fails. The young old, remaining silent about abuse may spring from an internalization of the pre-scription to remain independent and avoid being a burden on the public purse. Choosing silence may be one way to retain a positive social identity in the face of increasing ageism (Bytheway, 1995). The consequence may be extreme reluc-tance to seek assistance.

But when invited, older people do speak. In New South Wales, Australia, the Older Women Speak Up Project (Mears, 2003) set out to involve older women in documenting their experience of violence in interpersonal relationships in the home. The South Australian Older and Isolated Women and Domestic Violence Project (Schaeffer, 1999) commenced at the same time in South Australia. The incidence and lived experience of older people experiencing domestic violence was the focus of a third Australian study (Morgan Disney and Associates, 2000). Mears found that, 'despite the difficulties and the shame, older women will speak up about the violence in their lives if they are given a safe space and opportunity to do so and if they can expect to be believed' (2003: 1488). Ensuring a 'safe space' may require ensuring the permission of the society: she found that many women who shared their accounts of violence had lived with the effects of vio-lence for their entire lives – 'for 70, 80 and even 90 years – and most had never spoken about these experiences'. It was now possible for them to do so.

As the World Health Organization and the International Network for the Prevention of Elder Abuse found, when conducting a large, international study of older people's perception of abuse, this is not universally possible. This ground breaking study (WHO and INPEA, 2002), which set out to challenge existing def-initions of elder abuse, sought the views of older people (defined as 60 years and over) and primary healthcare workers in eight countries on abuse – how they clas-sified it and how they perceived 'the first steps needed for a global strategy' (2002: 1).

Primarily this study challenged the 'individualistic focus' of the elder abuse lit-erature, its emphasis on pathology (of victims, perpetrators, families) and empha-sized 'structural-societal factors' (2002: 8). Six key categories were identified by participants:

- Structural and societal abuse, identified by many as the primary kind of abuse causing most of the other types of abuse and linked by participants to governments' failure to provide basic services.
- Neglect and abandonment, for example of older people at hospitals in countries like Kenya and Brazil, and linked with seasonal conditions.
- Disrespect and ageist attitudes, which are described as pervasive, including in healthcare systems.
- Psychological, emotional and verbal abuse.
- Physical abuse, sometimes a difficult form of abuse to be named, particularly in India, where the words could not be used.
- Legal and financial abuse, for instance abuse of dowry laws in India, and inheritance laws in Lebanon.

Underpinning virtually all forms and contexts of abuse were gender and socio-economic status.

It is clear that any approach to the problem of 'elder abuse' must start with acknowledging that it is sourced in the social and structural arrangements of all societies. It is an issue of inequality and injustice. It is clear that it is not possible for all who experience and live with it to name it. But living in safety is surely a human right. How, if at all, can a rights framework address the common and very different circumstances inhabited by older people, both within and across countries?

Implications for human service professionals

The documents produced by the Economic and Social Council and the World Health Organization are consistent with each other in elaborating how human rights frameworks can translate into practice, guided by zero tolerance of violation of fundamental human rights. Both lay store on awareness and education – education of older people themselves about their rights as well as about abuse, of professions, media and communities. Both affirm a proper place for 'Legislation, protective mechanisms and legal intervention … legal structures to penalize violence, that can address the mistreatment of older persons, are important to uphold' (Commission for Social Development, UN, 2002: 8). Prevention and intervention are conceptualized together (Commission for Social Development, UN, 2002a: 9). And specifically defined rights-based interventions are embedded in a call for efforts to address broad structural inequalities, particularly poverty.

We do not naively assume that the production of policy documents of themselves change situations of inequality and injustice. Political will and courage, availability of financial, material, information and education resources, must follow the claims that older people are now being sufficiently courageous to make. The redundancy and discrimination felt by older people in a world of increasing social mobility and inequality, of individualism and privatization will continue while limits to growth are ignored. It is sometimes said that older people are feared, and their claim to equal rights dismissed, because they remind us of the fact that life has limits; for all of us life ends. We all die, usually now in old age. What kind of end-of-life is everyone entitled to? The Research Agenda on Ageing for the 21st Century (Commission for Social Development, 2002b) names elder abuse, neglect, violence and exploitation as a specific topic in the critical research arena 'Social Participation and Integration'. The evidence in this chapter demonstrates that it is imperative to engage in such research.

Chapter summary

Older people and violence

- Violence towards older people has been described in terms of elder abuse.
- The response to elder abuse has been driven by professionals.

(Continued)

- Understanding of the social position of older people in the twenty-first century must start within an appreciation of ageism.
- Older people experiencing violence and oppression have been described in different ways related to how violence has been explained.
- Current approaches to elder abuse emphasize the social, structural and systemic reasons and therefore requiring multi-level responses.
- Older people themselves are now identifying their perceptions of the kinds of violence that they wish to address. This does not always accord with professionals' views.
- Recent research points to the need both for gender to centrally inform understandings and for domestic violence and elder abuse services to collaborate more closely with each other.
- However defined, harmful acts towards older people are abusive of fundamental human rights.
- Underpinning virtually all forms and contexts of abuse were gender and socio-economic status.

16 Human service professionals, violence and the workplace

Rosalie Pockett

The workplace: a microcosm of society

Just as the 'market' can be defined as anywhere there is a buyer, a seller and a product, the 'workplace' can similarly be defined as anywhere there is an employer, an employee and a product. It is both the conceptual and actual location of industry, bringing together members of society for broadly defined economic activity.

However, the *social* significance of the workplace lies beyond the economic view of labour, capital, employer and employee coming together in specific relationships. The workplace reflects the values and beliefs of individuals and of society and these underpin the human endeavour. Thus 'the workplace' can be considered a microcosm of the wider society in which it exists. Workplace relationships may be affected by workers' beliefs and experiences around issues of gender, class, religion, ethnicity and sexuality. For example, a study of workplace experiences of gay men, lesbians and transgender people concluded, 'Homophobic harassment and prejudicial treatment spanned all occupations, industries and types and sizes of the employing organizations' (Irwin, 1999: 6).

Violence and abuse within the workplace context has received lesser attention than debates concerning domestic violence and family violence. Reasons for this include the perception that the workplace has been a relatively safe and violence-free environment (Chappell and Di Martino, 2000). Since the late 1990s however, international events such as the Dunblane massacre in the United Kingdom and Port Arthur in Australia have been identified not only as mass casualty events, but also incidents of violence that occurred within the workplace.

It could also be argued that the priority of feminist perspectives has been to relocate violence against women and children from the private to the public domain focusing on the development of public policy in this context. For further discussion on this see Chapter 6, 'Feminism(s) and domestic violence within national policy contexts'. It might also be argued that workplaces (unlike families and personal relationships), were already considered to be in the public domain as legislation, regulation and public policy already existed for many aspects of worker/work/ workplace relationships. However, these arguments are contested and can be challenged on the basis of gendered perspectives that exist in public policy.

It is only within the last decade that violence and abuse in the workplace has been named as a workplace issue within the context of the broader feminist debates of violence and intimate partner relationships. In a retrospective study of workplace homicides over a fifteen year period in the American state of North Carolina, 75 per cent of female homicides in 'dispute-related homicides' in the workplace occurred in the context of an estranged intimate relationship. This was in significant contrast with data gathered on male 'dispute-related homicides' where the dispute was most likely to be work related (Moracco, Runyan and Loomis, 2000). Similarly, domestic disputes that were carried over and acted out in the workplace were both higher in number, and of greater significance for employers and managers, than the more usually anticipated incidents between employees (Scalora, Washington and Casady, 2003).

This chapter will undertake a critical analysis of violence and human service professionals in the workplace. It will explore a number of contested debates such as the incidence, measurement and costs of workplace violence, the causative factors and the current discourse on the management, containment and elimination of workplace violence. It will also identify areas requiring further study.

Defining the 'workplace' for human service professionals

Within the scope of this chapter, the workplace can be defined in two different ways. First, by the organizational context, that defines the human service professional as 'an employee'. The majority of human service professionals are employed in either the public or government sector, or in the community and NGO (non-government organization) sector, and these sectors can be collectively described in the workplace as 'the employers'. In the context of this definition, violence is referred to as 'workplace' violence. The second approach is to define the workplace by the practice context that defines the human service professional as a 'professional practitioner'. This approach includes an understanding of the values, ethics, skills, and intervention of the practitioner with their client/s that define professional practice, autonomy and responsibility. In the context of this definition, violence is referred to as 'occupational' violence.

Within these two contexts, as employees and as professional practitioners, human service professionals may have similar roles including those of service providers, agents of care and control, work colleagues and citizens.

Definitions of violence and abuse in the workplace

The naming and defining of violence is a social process which is linked to the position or relationship of the person to the violent activity or behaviour (Hearn, 1996). Definitions of workplace violence have traditionally been located in the industrial discourse of occupational health and safety, workers' rights and risk management. These definitions are internationally consistent and by including concepts of both violence and abuse, a broader range of behaviours has been identified. For example two definitions of workplace violence are:

any incident in which an individual is abused, threatened or assaulted and includes verbal, physical or psychological abuse, threats or other intimidating behaviours, intentional physical attacks, aggravated assault, threats with an offensive weapon, sexual harassment and sexual assault.

(NSW Health, 2005: 4)

incidents where employees are abused, threatened, assaulted or subject to other offensive behaviour in circumstances related to their work.

(Di Martino and Musri, 2001: 7)

Occupational violence has been defined as:

The attempt or actual exercise by a person of any force so as to cause injury to a worker, including any threatening statement or behaviour which gives a worker reasonable cause to believe he or she is at risk.

(National Occupational Health and Safety Commission
[NOHSC], 1999: 1)

Consistent with the interpretative approach to abuse and violence discussed by Hearn, workplace violence has many facets and its complexity lends itself to critical analysis to understand both its construction and the consequent ways it may be managed and addressed in the workplace. Contemporary understanding of violence at work is that it is a complex interaction of individual, structural and contextual factors.

The manifestations of violence in the workplace

Existing literature on workplace violence has classified incidents into four main categories although differences exist in the location of some incidents in each category (Mayhew and Chappell, 2001; Bowie, 2002). These four categories comprise: client initiated violence; external violence; internal violence or relationship violence; and organizational violence and systemic violence. Each of these will be outlined in turn.

Client initiated violence

This is traditionally the most commonly described workplace violence experienced by human service professionals and the majority of the earliest literature focused on this category. Particular client groups and work contexts were identified as carrying higher risks of exposure to incidents of this nature, for example, working with involuntary clients; in child protection; and with victims of domestic violence. Exposure to violent situations vicariously, that is, through the client or the situation, was also identified as a type of workplace violence for human service professionals (Sayers, 1986; Bibby, 1994; Puckett and Cleak, 1994; Dekel and Peled, 2000; Way, VanDeusen, Martin, Applegate and Jandle, 2004; Tehrani, 2004). Within the category of client initiated violence, distinctions have been made by human service professionals according to the perceived level of clients' individual responsibility for the behaviour. A client with a mental illness for example, who is aggressive towards a practitioner may be perceived and treated quite differently from a client who is responsible for their actions and acts aggressively with deliberate intent. Despite the differing perceptions by the human service professional, the incident itself is still statistically viewed as an incident of workplace violence.

External violence

Incidents in this category include violence inflicted by others from outside the workplace on employees, for example, a bomb threat or armed hold up. Bowie (2002) includes terrorist acts in this category, however other authors have identified this as a separate category of 'intentional violence', which is defined as violence inflicted on civilians by others with political, religious or ideological motives (Boscarino, Figley and Adams, 2004).

Internal violence or relationship violence

This occurs between employees within a workplace. This may be either between employees at the same level of the organization, sometimes referred to as 'horizontal violence' or between supervisor and supervisee for example bullying and harassment (Duffy, 1995; Spring and Stern, 1998, 1999). This type of violence includes such behaviours as threats of termination, 'official' reprisals and intimidatory and threatening behaviour.

Domestic violence or intimate partner violence that is brought to the workplace is also included in this category. Within this category similarities have been identified between the features of domestic violence or intimate partner violence, and workplace bullying. These features include power relationships between the victim (the subordinate worker) and the perpetrator (the manager or supervisor); the inability of the victim to leave the situation; and the frequency and opportunity of contact. The long term psychological impact of workplace bullying has been recognized as being similar to that of other long term abusive relationships (Leymann 1990; Roberts, 2000; Tehrani, 2004).

Both horizontal violence and relationship violence involve the interaction of personal power and oppression. The subordination of another continues the personal cycle of abuse within the workplace context.

Organizational violence and systemic violence

A further typology of 'organizational violence' derived from the third category, has been suggested by Bowie (2002). Incidents of this nature may occur as a result of the operational, procedural or policy aspects of the organization as a service provider or as an employer. It may be argued that human service professionals, as employees, may be participants in oppressive practices of the agency, towards clients and service recipients. It may be further argued that practitioners have a professional responsibility to practise in an anti-oppressive way, and ensure that systemic abuse of clients is prevented. In taking action however, they may become identified as 'troublesome' for the organization. Public interest disclosures or 'whistleblowing' has been identified as a causative factor in 'official reprisals' and abusive behaviour towards individual staff (De Maria and Jan, 1994; De Maria, 1996). Despite political support and enactment of various forms of whistleblower legislation to protect workers the subtleties of abuse by intimidation and other covert means remain (Hoffman, 2006).

The intersection of workplace and occupation violence: experiences from practice

---

Case example

A social work student at a Social Services office had an appointment made in her diary to see 'Katy'. The reason for the referral was 'housing issues, needs to talk to social worker directly'. English was not Katy's first language and she was accompanied to the appointment by her son aged ten and her brother-in-law who acted as an interpreter. Katy had four children and along with her brother-in-law were on temporary resident visas and thus not eligible for public housing.

Katy was in the early stages of labour in the waiting room but her brother-in-law insisted that they wait to see the social worker. The social worker suggested that Katy go immediately to hospital but her brother-in-law began to raise his voice insisting that the interview proceed. The social work student's account of what then followed –

> Once we sat down around the table in the interview room, Katy's brother-in-law asked me why I wanted to see Katy. I understood that this was a client initiated request ... Katy's brother-in-law abruptly advised that 'some social worker called us last week and told us to come here, and then someone will give us a house'. I explained that Social Services did not arrange housing and that this was done by the Department of Housing.
>
> [The social work student continues] ... this sparked a wild reaction from him. 'What do you mean you can't give me any housing ... you people told my sister-in-law to come here, and then we will get a house ... Can't you see she is about to give birth ... why do you put us in this situation? ... we are not leaving until you give us a house!'

Sensing that this was moving beyond her abilities, the social work student advised them that she would seek advice from her supervisor. The supervisor

---

> *(Continued)*
>
> found out more details and in fact a staff member had contacted them last week by phone to give them information about the Department Housing. Both the student and the supervisor were now in the room and the information was given to the brother-in-law. The brother-in-law exploded into anger, shouting and yelling. Katy was now in labour and needed hospital care immediately. The situation had turned into a disaster. Finally one of the staff activated the alarm to indicate that an incident was occurring and that security and the Police may be needed.
>
> (Example courtesy of Grace Ye, 2006)

This situation would undoubtedly be registered as a violent workplace incident; however, in using a singular typology the inherent underpinnings that mitigate the situation are not recognized. Neither is the systemic violence towards the client recognized. Exploring the case study from a theoretical perspective the final violent outburst is likely to be a result of the interplay of several key factors including the failure of social policy in making provision for the social support needs of temporary residents (see Chapter 11, 'Violence and the state: asylum seeker children'); bureaucratic processes that conflict and overlap with one another; the subservience of Katy's needs to patriarchy within the family unit and the individual psychology of frustration and anger. This may have been compounded by the inexperience of the workers involved.

Zero tolerance policies and procedures, and the use of 'incident review' tools such as root cause analysis, often mitigate against the process of seeking knowledge about the underlying causes. They may also revert to blaming individual workers and contribute to the sense of failure and unease by staff that a situation could have been avoided (Puckett and Cleak, 1994; Bowie, 2002).

Measuring workplace violence: international comparisons

In a comprehensive report on violence in the workplace commissioned by the International Labour Office, workplace bullying was identified as one of the fastest growing forms of workplace violence with women workers experiencing higher levels of bullying than male workers (Chappell and Di Martino, 2000; Tehrani, 2004). Other forms of workplace violence included physical assault, homicide, robbery, sexual assault and intimidatory behaviours such as victimizing, ostracizing, innuendo and deliberate silence.

The definition of workplace violence and the subset of behaviours that may be included are problematic however, as a result of the extensive range of behaviours that can potentially fall into this category, and the concomitant qualification that may occur around the behaviour as a result of individual and cultural norms around acceptability.

Since the variety of behaviours which may be covered under the general rubric of violence at work is so large, the borderline with acceptable behaviours is often so vague, and the perception in different contexts and cultures of what constitutes violence is so diverse, it becomes a significant challenge to both describe and define this phenomenon.

(Mayhew and Chappell, 2001: 397)

Similarly, data about workplace and occupational violence is not readily available nor empirically comparable (Mayhew and Chappell, 2001). The incidence of violence in the workplace in Britain has been falling steadily since 1995 where 1.3 million incidents were reported. The British Crime Survey (2004/5) estimated the figure to be 50 per cent lower at 665,000. The majority of these incidents were defined as 'client initiated' violence. This figure is reported as low with violent incidents at work being classified as 'rare'. However, in terms of occupational violence, police, social workers, probation officers, publicans and bar staff, security guards, nurses and other health staff, transport workers and community youth workers were most at risk of violence at work (Budd, 1999). The situation in the United Kingdom is comparable to that in Australia and the United States of America. The work practices of some occupations place professionals in situations of greater risk, for example the activity of home visiting with a client by a social worker or other human service professional may be translated into the generic high risk activity of 'transporting a stranger in a car' (Bibby, 1994).

Despite the lack of consistent empirical data, the incidence of risk of violence in both the workplace and occupational groups that include human service professionals is increasing. A comprehensive international literature review on occupational violence has drawn a number of conclusions about the risks of exposure to workplace violence. The highest risk of external violence is in workplaces where money or drugs are handled. Client initiated violence is a common experience for workers who have a high degree of face-to-face contact with clients and their families and internal violence within organizations is most common where 'dominant/subordinate hierarchical relationships exist' (Mayhew and Chappell, 2001: 14). Given that the work of human service professionals can fall into all three of these categories, it can be surmised that the risk of exposure of human service professionals to workplace violence is quite high.

The economic costs of workplace violence

The imprecise nature of determining the costs of violence and stress at work, and the economic benefits of a 'violence-free' and 'stress-free' working environment, has led to the conclusion that data in this area is unreliable and requiring considerable qualification. A lack of clarity and consistency exists between the concepts of 'direct' costs such as sick leave absences, which can be measured in monetary terms, and 'indirect costs' such as the human cost of stress-related illnesses (Hoel, Sparks and Cooper, 2001). Citing examples from a number of industrialized nations, Hoel and colleagues argue that health insurance costs to employers have risen significantly as a direct result of employee stress-related claims. In a study of 5,000 hospital staff in Finland those staff that had been bullied had 26 per cent more certified sickness absence than those who were not, with the authors indicating that the figures were probably an underestimation of the situation (Kivimäki, Elovainio and Vathera, 2000). In Australia, the findings in a report commissioned by the Office for the Status of Women in 2004, indicated that the total annual cost of domestic violence in 2002–3 was approximately $AUD 8.1billion (Access Economics, 2004). Conclusions can be drawn from this report about the costs of violence within the workplace.

Explaining workplace violence: causative factors of workplace violence

Despite differing definitions, one of the fundamental principles which has under-pinned the more traditional debates explaining workplace violence has been that of the causative factors for workplace violence. An early study undertaken by the Tavistock Institute of Human Relations in the United Kingdom recognized the interactional nature of violence:

> The problem may lie in the assailant, in that there may be something about him which makes him strike out an employee. The employee may be partly to blame because of incompetence or because of an unsympathetic attitude, or the way the organization works may sometimes lead to misunderstanding or frustration.
>
> (Poynter and Warne, 1988: 399)

Psychological and behavioural theories that examine violence as a manifestation of aggression can also be used to understand the causative factors of incidents. For example, behavioural theory suggests that aggression is a learned behaviour and ecological and sociological theories explain aggression as a result of the circumstances of surroundings, context and roles (Braithwaite, 2001). Whilst these theories attempt to explain the relationship between the individual and their environment as factors, Bowie (2002) has suggested that the interactions of the various typologies of workplace violence mentioned earlier may also shed light on potential causative factors.

The abusive dominance of one group over another in the workplace is another manifestation of violence. Oppressive interactions between individuals and groups in the workplace may lead to hardship and injustice (Thompson, 2006). Examining workplace violence from this perspective may help to understand the suspected high level of under-reporting of workplace incidents (Mayhew and Chappell, 2001). Reasons for workers not reporting incidents of bullying include the belief that it would not be taken seriously; that it would make matters worse; and that the perpetrator of the bullying was also the manager or supervisor (Rains, 2001; Tehrani, 2004). This perspective is also useful in the analysis of workplace abuse experienced by particular groups of workers characterized by social exclusion.

Theories of oppression would explain this as the denial of citizenship (Thompson, 2006). Indigenous workers may experience both racial oppression within the workplace and professional oppression. For more detail see Chapter 5, 'Towards healing: recognizing the trauma surrounding Aboriginal family violence'. The latter has been identified by those workers in Indigenous specific roles such as Aboriginal health workers and includes a lack of acceptance of the qualifications and skills of Indigenous workers.

> For Aboriginal health workers, the double jeopardy is that although these laws (Occupational Health and Safety) are in place to protect them, they are normally so disempowered and disillusioned by these behaviours not only in the workplace but also from the Aboriginal community in which they work and live that there is not a preparedness, formal expression or strength to carry through with the complaint system.
>
> (Winsor, 2001: 7)

The relationship between workplace violence and workplace stressors: the human and economic costs of managerialism

Definitions of workplace 'stress' have identified the interaction of the individual worker with inadequate job definition, a lack of clarity in structure and inadequate resources (Di Martino and Musri, 2001). A study of social workers in teaching hospitals in Australia identified workplace stresses that contributed to the understanding of the occupational culture of hospital social work and the effect of this on the turnover of the social work workforce. Hospitals were often identified by social work participants in the study as abusive and competitive environments. To work effectively, social workers needed particular skills to negotiate the organizational and bureaucratic relationships in hospitals. The workplace stresses of a burdensome, demanding organization combined with a lack of adequate resources were identified by social workers as being of greater significance to their levels of job satisfaction and decisions to stay or leave the job, than the demands of complex cases and client work (Pockett, 2003).

The elimination of causative factors that may lead to workplace violence has been identified as a responsibility of the employer and an indicator of effective management. However, it may be argued that there is a growing perceived relationship between the impact of managerialism itself, within a neo-conservative ideology, and the increasing prevalence of bullying and harassment in the workplace. In an audit tool for nursing, a number of workplace characteristics were identified as potential stressors or risks. These included poor communication, poor task environment and a poor problem solving environment (Cox and Griffith, 1994). The existence of a direct relationship between organizational change, demanding workloads, a negative work environment and the increasing incidence of bullying in the workplace, has also been suggested (Hoel *et al.*, 2001). It may also be argued that the current management hegemony itself is a significant contributing factor.

The dominance of the managerial approach manifests itself in another important way that affects social workers. When things are not working, or there are problems, the inevitable managerial response is either to bring in yet more managers or to institute an organizational restructure, in the belief that problems are best solved through organizational change. Hence social workers find themselves working in an almost constantly changing environment of restructuring and organizational 'development' with the corresponding problems of uncertainty, insecurity and low morale.

(Ife, 1997: 18)

Given the changing emphasis in the work/leisure balance in the industrialized world as a result of economic imperatives, and the existence of smaller, older and less regulated workforces, it is likely that significant quality of life issues will spillover into the workplace in the twenty-first century. It is expected that the indirect costs of longer working hours on interpersonal relationships will also have a longer-term impact on relationships in the workplace (Peetz, 2006). The impact on employee turnover and workforce retention in workplaces that are perceived as being abusive to employees will be significant. These trends require further study.

Preventing and containing workplace violence: safety and organizational risk management

In contemporary practice, human service professionals are usually introduced to the concept of 'workplace violence' as a potential risk within the scope of occupational health and safety requirements of their employing agency. The incidence of occupational health and safety legislation, policies and procedures grew out of a convergence of a number of factors evident in the last two decades of the twentieth century. These factors included the long held collectivist views about worker safety expressed by unions, recognition of the burden of costs to employers of workers' compensation programmes and the wider economic costs of injured workers out of the workplace, and the emergence of anti-discrimination legislation that preserved and protected workers from an individual rights perspective.

The conflation of these factors was underpinned by both the common law and statutory law around the duty of care of employers to employees. Within occupational health and safety legislation, the responsibilities of employers and employees were included. Within the workplace, employers have a legal responsibility to provide a safe workplace and to ensure that risks to staff are prevented where possible. Employees have a reciprocal responsibility to participate in the assessment of risk of harm and to follow agreed safe work practices. These activities are undertaken as risk control and management strategies. Other strategies include conflict resolution, grievance procedures and stress management. It has been argued that such strategies, within this discourse, may identify the worker as the problem (Bowie, 2002).

The occupational health and safety lexicon has become the dominant discourse around violence in the workplace. It may be argued that female dominated professions particularly in the health and social care sectors (for example nursing), have elevated workplace violence to a legitimate workplace hazard through targeted Zero Tolerance campaigns (NSW Health, 2005). However, it may also be argued that such campaigns may have the effect of denying or closing off legitimate complaints and grievances (Bowie, 2002).

It may also be argued that horizontal violence exists between occupational groups and is based on the oppression of one group over another.

> To my surprise a lot of these articles [about horizontal violence] were written on or on behalf of nurses who claimed to be the victims of oppression by doctors ... from my experience it was the nurses and other health professionals, who in general are the oppressors of Aboriginal health workers ... the oppressed become the oppressors – the cycle of turning the frustration inward on your own or someone that you see as 'lower' than yourself.
>
> (Winsor-Dahlstrom, 2000: 82)

It may also be argued that the effect of this mainstream lexicon has resulted in workplace violence being discussed in a 'non-gendered' way with little reference to issues of power, roles and the voices of individual experience (Office of Women, 2006). If, as this study found, women in the workforce have difficulty naming aspects of behaviour as abusive or intimidatory, the silent voices of more marginalized groups in the workforce are yet to be heard (Bell, 2003; Brown, Puller and Bradley, 2006). With regard to the Indigenous workforce, several studies have included Indigenous workers in participant samples (Irwin, 1999; Office of Women's Policy, 2005); however targeted studies on workplace violence and Indigenous workers are required.

Implications for human service professionals

In contemporary practice, human service professionals may find themselves responding to acts of external violence or intentional violence in a professional capacity as service providers, but, at the same time, they may be members of the community that has been threatened or attacked. For example, an incident may occur on such a large scale that it is classified as a disaster, such as an airplane crash or train crash; or maybe as a result of an intentional act of violence that in contemporary literature may be called an act of terrorism. Each of these incidents may result in mass casualties where the social worker or human service professional is both a member of the community in which the event has taken place as well as a service provider to those affected by the disaster:

> When helping professionals share the same traumatic event with their clients, multiple levels of vulnerability to traumatisation emerge in working with

survivors. ... This condition is particularly challenging when helpers are confronted by the realization that they are part of the attacked community.

(Somer, Buchbinder, Peled-Avram and Ben-Yzhack, 2004: 1077, 1087)

Workplaces made up of 'first responder' professionals should have programmes in place that support the behavioural, cognitive and emotional domains of workers' responses to the violent incident (Fraidlin and Rabin, 2006). Emerging from the literature on disaster management, a number of strategies have been established using critical incident stress management approaches. Sustaining and supporting the workforce in self-care activities and peer support were identified as priorities following exposure to violent or critical incidents. Such strategies are based on an understanding of human resilience and survivorship. Workplace violence of this nature challenges both the personal and professional aspects of practice.

A study of violence in the social work workplace in Canada found that the majority of social workers interviewed reported experiencing some form of violence in their work; however four-fifths reported feeling safe or fairly safe in their work environment. The study also concluded,

> that social workers may have difficulty talking about client violence, because in so doing they may feel they are contributing to the oppression that their clients experience as a result of inequities of our social and economic structure and by virtue of their clients' age, race, ethnicity, gender class, sexual orientation and physical or mental ability.

(MacDonald and Sirotich, 2005: 778)

The 'relationship' aspect of the worker–client relationship is identified as being significant in the willingness or otherwise of the worker to report incidents of violence.Reporting incidents may betray the collaborative partnership that workers try to establish with clients, and yet working with some clients makes social workers both emotionally and physically vulnerable. A sense of failure, guilt, incompetence, and an inability to continue to work has been reported by social workers who experienced client violence (Puckett and Cleak, 1994; Bibby, 1994; Jayaratne, Vinokur-Kaplan, Nagda and Chess, 1996).

Human service professionals will continue to be part of the workforce as employees and as professional practitioners. These givens co-exist with the ambiguities and contradictions inherent in this dual relationship. Extraordinary events narrowly defined by traditional modernity can create problems for the professional practitioner in finding effective strategies for intervention, enabling the voices of the disadvantaged to be heard. Human service professionals, as professional practitioners, must understand the construction of the abuse or violence. This is often a confronting challenge when they are also participants in the workplace experience (Riley, 1996). The experience of abuse and violence may be a personal one raising many dilemmas and challenges for practice. A well-trained workforce needs to incorporate the technical rationality of safety with the ability to practice in a critically reflective way. This is the responsibility of all human service professionals.

Chapter summary

Human service professionals, violence and the workplace

- The existence of workplace violence is not contested; however the reporting of workplace violence incidents has occurred within the occupational health and safety discourse.
- Internationally, differences and inconsistencies exist in definitions and measurement of workplace violence and there are contested debates around the incidence and causative factors of workplace violence.
- Human service professionals in the workforce are consistently identified in occupational classifications carrying high levels of risk and it is assumed that the incidence of 'under reporting' is quite high.
- It has been argued that contributing to this under reporting is the ability or otherwise of employees in the workplace, particularly those from more socially marginalized groups such as women, Indigenous workers, and gay, lesbian and transgender people, to name the abusive behaviour and to feel confident to report it without repercussions. The expectations around professional practice by human service professionals are also a factor.
- Areas for further study are identified including the intersection of domestic violence and the workplace, workplace violence and Indigenous workers, and the lexicon of workplace violence, public policy and gender.

17 Conclusion

Embarking on this book we wanted to provide practitioners and policy makers with material about the current debates and challenges regarding violence, abuse and oppression from an international perspective for different groupings in different contexts. What has ensued is a rich discussion on the implications for policy and practice where issues related to difference, diversity and complexity abound. The authors have adeptly woven together a number of arguments about violence, abuse and oppression; debated a diversity of definitional issues; considered different ways of understanding violence; raised numerous questions; summarized current research and highlighted its gaps and limitations.

The focus of each chapter and the range of issues covered all reflect the need to be open to diversity and difference when considering current debates and challenges about violence, abuse and oppression. Three key themes resonate throughout the book. First is the understanding that violence, abuse and oppression is multi-faceted and complex, intersecting with age, ethnicity, indigenous issues, class, level of physical or mental ability and sexuality, as well as structural factors such as poverty and entrenched historical disadvantage. The need to respect human rights and the meaningful participation of all citizens has been highlighted as being central to addressing violence, abuse and oppression. Second is the importance of taking into account gender as the implications of gendered power imbalances feature significantly in many of the chapters and issues of power and responsibility and what is heard and what is not heard is integral to all discussions relating to these areas. Third are the implications for human service professionals which feature in the final sections of each chapter. Influencing this third area are the professionals' own experiences and understandings of violence in the workplace. We review these key themes in relation to responses to violence, abuse and oppression, consider resource issues, highlight the messages for human service professionals and suggest possible ways forward.

Responses to violence and oppression

Each of the chapters in this book has highlighted a number of different areas that need to be addressed in response to violence against the particular group or policy intervention in question. The responses are dependent upon the ways in which violence, abuse and oppression and underlying assumptions about rights and responsibilities are viewed. Feminist perspectives and public health and risk discourses have underpinned the development of the responses in a number of the chapters. In addition, human rights discourse are central, either implicitly or explicitly, to all groups, where the needs and rights of all citizens not to be subject to violence, abuse and oppression has formed the basic tenet for all strategies. Ideally, these strategies are based on inclusive policies and practices and socially just laws implemented through welfare, social, health and legal services. The strategies include community education, professional education, community development, prevention programmes, early intervention, crisis intervention, statutory activity, legal action and recovery programmes. Throughout all these strategies what is required is a comprehensive response where the voices of those experiencing violence are central to the action taken. In this way professionals can be alerted to not only the needs of all parties but also gain knowledge about the possible unintended consequences of particular interventions.

Allocation of adequate resources

One of the major stumbling blocks to responding to violence, abuse and oppression in the community is the allocation of adequate resources to address it. For instance, without adequate funding and coordination for essential programmes it is difficult for people living in poverty to weigh up their options for escaping violence. Similarly putting all one's eggs into one basket, such as focusing only on the legal response at the expense of general advocacy and support services for women can result in women being further abused by the legal system. Also if there are insufficient funds then allocation can become a competitive process with some groups missing out. Safety planning has to be prioritized, although, as noted in the chapter on disability and violence, the intentional or unintentional association of 'safety' with external control, can create further difficulties and reconfigure and compound abusive situations. Substantial resourcing of Aboriginal self-directed strategies is also crucial if the oppressive history and ongoing traumatic effects of assimilation policies and practices are to be effectively addressed. Additionally, as highlighted in the chapter on men and violence, funding allocation has to take into account the different requirements and claims of different individuals and groupings and to accept that, for example, safety planning for women and children, has to include work with violent men.

Messages for human service professionals

Multiple messages for human service professionals have been provided throughout this book. To summarize they include the:

- need for an increased emphasis on human rights;
- importance of deconstructing taken-for-granted assumptions about the operation of cultural, social and political power/knowledge frameworks;

- need to recognize and challenge existing institutional abuse and prevent future institutional abuse;
- importance of safety planning which operates from the perspective of those involved;
- necessity of safety planning for women and children including work with violent men;
- development of policies and practices which recognize the complexity and diversity of the lives of those who experience violence, abuse and oppression;
- provision of education and training for professionals about the complexity and diversity relating to violence in all groups;
- tackling of invisibility where violence, abuse and oppression is not recognized;
- challenging of heteronormative assumptions;
- foregrounding the perspectives of oppressed and marginalized groups and advocating for change and the resources to address these;
- constant review of support services to ensure that they are accessible and relevant;
- importance of working in partnership with those subject to violence, abuse and oppression;
- importance of acknowledging the harm that has been inflicted on Aboriginal people and the need to establish genuine partnerships incorporating the principle of Aboriginal self-determination;
- recognition of the resilience and skills of individuals and families;
- provision of assistance in increasing collaboration and the strengthening of informal support networks;
- adoption of flexible approaches in responding to unexpected challenges and unintended consequences;
- identification and fostering of strengths in challenging oppressive practices;
- recognition of the need for time for critical reflection and professional development;
- need for adequate support for human service workers who confront crisis and trauma on a regular basis; and
- need to provide sustaining and supporting self-care activities and peer support for workers, following exposure to violent or critical incidents.

Ways forward

Many ideas about future research and ways forward have been referred to throughout this book. These are key to developing further understandings and future policies and practices which are responsive to the voices of those who experience violence, abuse and oppression. Examples of suggested avenues for attention include ensuring that child welfare interventions and refugee policies actively generate and support the formation and operation of significant and flexible health and social support systems. Emphasis can also be placed on moving beyond legal responses to domestic violence and critically reflecting on the operation of power between perpetrator and victim, between women in different social locations, between women seeking help and those responding, and between the many agencies that are involved in intervening. Attention can also be paid to exploring the ways in which gendered power imbalances foster intimate partner violence in some contexts but not in others and examining how this can be explored without invoking traditional pathologizing explanations.There is additionally a need for an increased in-depth knowledge about the complexities of violence in lesbian relationships, particularly how the personal, social and political contexts influence how women experience violence in their lives. Similarly, the silencing that takes place in relation to older women and men has to be given priority so that the factors that contribute to oppressive experiences can be explored and addressed. Rural perspectives, the needs of those who consider violence against the self or suicide, the collective experiences of consumer/survivor movements, have also to be fully acknowledged in policy and practice arenas.

Ways forward also include a focus on practice research so that evidence about what works, how and why and in what circumstances, including location and culture, can be teased out so that the suitability and applicability to other locations can be assessed, modified and implemented. It is also important to draw from the experience of a wide range of cultures and countries in addressing violence, abuse and oppression and to ensure that there is cross-fertilization of knowledge between different areas (including social, welfare, health, legal and economic fields). In this, aspects such as the strengthening of resilience and spirituality need to be fully taken into account. There is also clearly a need to be more creative in the ways that messages about innovative policies and practices that can be seen to have positive outcomes are both rolled out and further facilitated. In turn, organizational cultures need to offer support to human service professionals as a matter of right and not as a measure of last resort and professional accreditation bodies have to prioritize courses focusing on addressing violence, abuse and oppression in relation to all areas and all social groupings.

On a positive note, the increasing global response to domestic violence and other forms of violence, oppression and abuse can be seen to have created a valuable resource of strength for human service providers in this field. As more research is carried out, as more culturally specific services are developed and as more emphasis is placed on human rights, the potential for improving social policy interventions and service models across all countries is increasing. The challenge is to persuade governments to fully invest in these areas and for human service professionals to work in partnership with those experiencing forms of violence, abuse and oppression to produce sustainable solutions that build on individual and community strengths and resilience.

Bibliography

Aboriginal Child Sexual Assault Taskforce. (2006). *Breaking the Silence: Creating the Future, Addressing child sexual assault in Aboriginal communities in NSW*. Sydney: Attorney General's Department NSW.

Abu-Lughod, L. (2002). Do muslim women really need saving? Anthropological reflections on cultural relativism and its Others. *American Anthropologist, 104*(3), 783–90.

Access Economics. (2004). *The Cost of Domestic Violence to the Australian Economy: Part 1 and Part 11*: Access Economics and Partnerships Against Domestic Violence (Australia). Canberra: Commonwealth of Australia.

AIHW. (2007). *Child Protection Australia 2005–2006*. Canberra: Australian Institute of Health and Welfare.

AIHW, Al-Yaman, F., Van Doeland, M. and Wallis, M. (2006). Family violence among Aboriginal and Torres Strait Islander peoples: Cat. no. IHW 17. Retrieved 3 November 2006, from http://www.aihw.gov.au/publications/ihw/fvaatsip/fvaatsip.pdf

Ainsworth, F. (2002). Mandatory reporting of child abuse and neglect: does it really make a difference? *Child and Family Social Work, 7*, 57–63.

Akister, A. (2006). A systems approach: back to the future – response to Munro, E. (2005) 'A Systems Approach to Investigating Child Abuse Deaths', British Journal of Social Work, 35(4), 531–46. *British Journal of Social Work, 36*, 159–61.

Alaszewski, A. (1998). Risk in modern society. In A. Alaszewski, L. Harrison and J. Manthorpe (eds), *Risk, Health and Welfare*. Buckingham: Open University Press.

Alderson, P. (2003). *Institutional Rights and Rites: A Century of Childhood*. London: Institute of Education.

Aldgate, J. (1988). Work with children experiencing separation and loss: a theoretical framework. In J. Aldgate and J. Simmons (eds), *Direct Work with Children* (pp. 36–48). London: British Association for Adoption and Fostering.

Allegro, P. (1975). The strange and the familiar: the evolutionary potential of lesbianism. In G. Covina and L. Galana (eds), *The Lesbian Reader* (pp. 167–84). Oakland, CA: Amazon Press.

Alliance for Self-Determination. (2001). Principles for self-determination. Retrieved online, www.ohsu. edu/selfdetermination/principles.html, Disabilities Act of 1990, 42 U.S.C. (section) 12101 et seq. 15 December 2006.

Almeida, R.V., and Durkin, T. (1999). The cultural context model: therapy for couples with domestic violence. *Journal of Marital and Family Therapy, 25*, 313–24.

Almeida, R.V., Woods, R., Messineo, T., Font, R.J. and Heer, C. (1994). Violence in the lives of the racially and sexually different: a public and private dilemma. *Journal of Feminist Family Therapy, 5*(3/4), 99–126.

Alston, M. (1995). *Women on the Land – The Hidden Heart of Rural Australia*. Kensington: University of New South Wales Press.

Alston, M. (1997). Violence against women in rural context. *Australian Social Work, 50*(1), 15–22.

Alston, M. (2007). Globalisation, rural restructuring and health service delivery in Australia: Policy failure and the role of social work? *Health and Social Care in the Community, 15*(3), 195–202.

American Psychiatric Association. (1994). *Diagnostic and Statistical Manual of Mental Disorders* (4th edn). Washington, DC: American Psychiatric Association.

Amnesty International. (2004). *National Plan of Action to Eliminate Violence Against Women*: Amnesty International Australia.

Anderson, D.K. and Saunders, D.G. (2003). Leaving an abusive partner. An empirical review of predictors, the process of leaving, and psychological well-being. *Trauma, Violence and Abuse, 4*(2), 163–91.

Anderson, P. (2001). You don't belong here in Germany: On the social situation of refugee children in Germany. *Journal of Refugee Studies, 14*(2), 187–99.

Anonymous. (1990). My name is legion, for we are many: Diagnostics and the psychiatric client. *Social Work, 38*(2), 391–2.

Antrobus, P. (2004). *The Global Women's Movement*. London: Zed Books.

Appleby, M. (1995). *Suicide Awareness Training Manual*. Narellan, NSW: Rose Education.

Asia Pacific Migration Research Network (APMRN). (1996). *Migration Issues in the Asia Pacific*. Issues Paper from Australia. Available online: http://www.unesco.org/most/apmrnwp5.htm (accessed 23 January 2007).

Assembly, U.N.G. (1993). Declaration on the Elimination of Violence against Women. Retrieved 5 February 2007, from http://www.unhchr.ch/huridocda/huridoca.nsf/(Symbol)/A.RES.48.104.En? Opendocument

Atkinson, J. (1990). Violence in Aboriginal Australia: colonisation and gender, Part 2. *The Aboriginal and Torres Strait Islander Health Worker, 14*(3), 4–27.

Atkinson, J. (2002). *Trauma Trails, Recreating Song Lines: The Transgenerational Effects of Trauma in Indigenous Australia*. North Melbourne, Australia: Spinifex Press.

Aubrey, C. and Dahl, S. (2006). Children's voices: The views of vulnerable children on their service providers and the relevance of the services they receive. *British Journal of Social Work, 36*, 21–39.

Australian Council of Heads of Schools of Social Work. (2006). *We've boundless plains to share: The first report of the People's Inquiry into Detention*. Perth.

Australian Council of Social Service (ACOSS). (2005). *Submission to the Senate Community Affairs Committee Inquiry into The Employment and Workplace Relations (Welfare to Work) Bill*. Canberra: Commonwealth of Australia.

Australian Department of Immigration and Citizenship. (2007). Fact Sheet 64. Temporary Protection Visas.

Australian Department of Immigration and Multicultural Indigenous Affairs. (2004). Canberra, DIMIA. Available online: http://www.immi.gov.au (accessed 15 January 2004).

Australian Government (1961). *McClements Royal Commission into Callan Park Mental Hospital*. Canberra: Australian Government.

Australian Institute of Health and Welfare. (2006). Child Protection Australia, 2004–05, AIHW cat. no. CWS 26. *Child Welfare Series no. 38*. Retrieved 2007 April 22, from http://www.aihw.gov. au/publications/cws/cpa04-05/cpa04-05.pdf

Australian Productivity Commission. (ed.). (2003). Overcoming Indigenous Disadvantage: Key Indicators. *2003 Report of the Steering Committee for the Review of Government Service Provision.* Canberra: Commonwealth Government of Australia.

Bacchi, C. (1999a). *Women, Policy and Politics, The Construction of Policy Problems.* London: Sage Publications

Bacchi, C.L. (1999b). Domestic violence: Battered women or violent men. In *Women, Policy and Politics: The construction of policy problems* (pp. 164–80). London: Sage.

Bachman, R. (2003). *Violence Against Women: Synthesis of Research for Criminal Justice Policymakers.* Washington, DC: National Institute of Justice. Available from, http://www.olp. usdoj.gov/nij/vawprog/synthesis_list.html

Bachrach, L. (1988). Defining chronic mental illness: A concept paper. *Hospital and Community Psychiatry, 39,* 383–8.

Bagshaw, D. and Chung, D. (2000). Men, Women and Domestic Violence. Retrieved 7 February 2007, from http://ofw.facs.gov.au/downloads/pdfs/d_v/women_men_dv.pdf

Bagshaw, D., Chung, D., Couch, M., Lilburn, S. and Wadham, B. (2000). *Reshaping Responses to Domestic Violence – Executive Summary.* Canberra.

Baker, P. (1997). And I went back: Battered women's negotiation of choice. *Journal of Contemporary Ethnography, 26*(1), 55–74.

Baker-Miller, J. (1976). *Towards a New Psychology of Women.* Harmondsworth: Penguin.

Ball, W. and Charles, N. (2006). Feminist social movements and policy change: Devolution, childcare and domestic violence policies in Wales. *Women's Studies International Forum, 29*(2), 172–83.

Bamblett, M. (2004). Living and learning together: a celebration and appreciation of diversity. *Developing Practice, 13*(Winter), 29.

Barlow, J. (2006). Home visiting for parents of pre-school children in the UK. In C. McAuley, P.J. Pecora and W. Rose (eds), *Enhancing the Well-being of Children and Families through Effective Interventions* (pp. 70–81). London: Jessica Kingsley Publishers.

Barnes, M. (2002). 'Taking over the asylum'. A paper for the critical psychiatry network conference, Birmingham. Retrieved 24 November 2006 from http://www.critpsynet. freeuk.com/barnes.htm

Barnes, M. and Bowl, R. (2001). *Taking Over the Asylum – Empowerment and Mental Health.* Basingstoke: Palgrave.

Barry, K. (1979). *Female Sexual Slavery.* Englewood Cliffs, NJ: Prentice Hall.

Bassman, R. (2001). Whose reality is it anyway? Consumers/survivors/ex-patients can speak for themselves. *Journal of Humanistic Psychology, 41*(4), 11–35.

Batavia, A. (2002). Consumer direction, consumer choice, and the future of long-term care. *Journal of Disability Policy Studies, 12*(2), 67–77.

Bates, L.M., Schuler, S.R., Islam, F. and Islam, M.K. (2004). Socioeconomic factors and processes associated with domestic violence in rural Bangladesh. *International Family Planning Perspectives, 30*(4), 190–9.

Bauman, Z. (2001). *Seeking Safety in an Insecure World.* Cambridge: Polity Press.

Baumeister, R. (1990). Suicide as escape from self. *Psychological Review, 97,* 90–113.

Bayne Smith, M.E. (1996). *Race, Gender, and Health.* London: Sage.

Beck, U. (2000). Risk society revisited: Theory, politics and research programmes. In B. Adam, U. Beck and J. van Loon (eds), *The Risk Society and Beyond: Critical Issues for Social Theory* (pp. 211–29). London: Sage.

Beckwith, J.B. (1993). Gender stereotypes and mental health revisited. *Social Behavior and Personality, 21*(1), 85–8.

Begum, N. (1992). Disabled women and the feminist agenda. *Feminist Review, 40*, 70–84.

Begum, N., Hill, M. and Stevens, A. (eds). (1994). *Reflections: the Views of Black Disabled People on their Lives and Community Care Paper 32.3.* London: CCETSW.

Behrendt, L. (2003). *Achieving Social Justice: Indigenous Rights and Australia's Future.* Sydney: The Federation Press.

Belknap, J. and Potter, H. (2005). The trials of measuring the 'success' of domestic violence policies. *Criminology and Public Policy, 4*(3), 559–66.

Bell, H. (2003). Cycles within cycles: Domestic violence, welfare and low-wage work. *Violence Against Women, 9*(10), 1245–62.

Belsky, J. (1978). Three theoretical models of child abuse: A critical review. *Child Abuse and Neglect, 2*, 37–49.

Bennett, L., Goodman, L. and Dutton, M.A. (1999). Systemic obstacles to the criminal prosecution of a battering partner: A victim perspective. *Journal of Interpersonal Violence, 14*(7), 761–72.

Bentovim, A. (2006). Therapeutic intervention with children who have expereinced sexual and physical abuse in the UK. In C. McAuley, P.J. Pecora and W. Rose (eds), *Enhancing the Well-being of Children and Families through Effective Interventions. International Evidence for Practice* (pp. 143–57). London: Jessica Kingsley Publishers.

Beresford, P. (2004). 'Where's the evidence?' *Mental Health Today, Feb*, 31–4.

Beresford, Q. and Omaji, P. (1999). *Our State of Mind: Racial Planning and the Stolen Generations.* South Fremantle, Western Australia: Fremantle Arts Centre Press.

Bevacqua, M. and Baker, C. (2004). 'Pay no attention to the man behind the curtain!': Power, privacy, and the legal regulation of violence against women. *Women & Politics, 26*(3–4), 57–83.

Bhat, D. (2006). India's landmark Domestic Abuse Law comes into effect. *Times Online.* Retrieved 26 October 2006, from http://www.tomesonline.co.uk/article/ 0,25689-2422644,00.html

Bibby, P. (1994). *Personal Safety for Social Workers*: Suzy Lamplugh Trust, UK.

Biggs, S. (1993). *Understanding Ageing: Images, Attitudes and Professional Practice.* Buckingham and Philadelphia: Open University Press.

Biggs, S. (1995). *Elder Abuse in Perspective.* Buckingham and Philadelphia: Open University Press.

Biggs, S., Phillipson, C. and Kingston, P. (1995). *Elder Abuse in Perspective.* Buckingham: Open University Press.

Bird, C. (ed.). (1998). *The Stolen Generation: Their Stories.* Sydney: Random House.

Bird, K. (2004). Towards a feminist analysis of lesbian relationship violence II. *Home Truths: Stop Sexual Assault and Domestic Violence, a National Challenge.* Retrieved 11 December 2006, from http://www.hometruths.com.au/presentations/Bird_Towards_a_ Feminist_Analysis_of_Lesbian_Relationship_Violence.doc

Blaska, B. (1991). First person account: What it is like to be treated like a CMI. *Schizophrenia Bulletin, 17*, 172–76.

Bograd, M. (1999). Strengthening domestic violence theories: Intersections of race, class, sexual orientation, and gender. *Journal of Marital and Family Therapy, 25*(3), 275–89.

Boltz, S. (1992). *Creating Partnerships with Self-help: Differences in the Self-help and Professional roles* (Center for Self-Help Research, Working Paper series). Berkeley: CA: Center for Self-Help Research.

Boraine, A. (1997) *Statement made at the Australian Aboriginal Reconciliation Convention, Melbourne.*

Boscarino, J., Figley, C. and Adams, R. (2004). Compassion fatigue following the September 11 terrorist attacks: A study of secondary trauma among New York City social workers. *International Journal of Emergency Mental Health*, 6(2), 57–66.

Bosch, K. and Schumm, W.R. (2004). Accessibility to resources: Helping rural women in abusive partner relationships become free from abuse. *Journal of Sex & Marital Therapy*, 30(5), 357–70.

Bowie, V. (1996). *Coping with Violence: a Guide for the Human Services*. London: Whiting and Birch.

Bowie, V. (1998). *Workplace Violence*. Paper presented at the Australian Institute of Criminology Conference, Crime Against Business, Melbourne, Victoria.

Bowie, V. (2002). Workplace violence. Sydney: Workcover New South Wales Government.

Bowlby, J. (1988). *A Secure Base: Parent–Child Attachment and Healthy Human Development*. New York Basic Books.

Bracken, P. and Thomas, P. (2005). *Postpsychiatry*. Oxford: Oxford University Press.

Braithwaite, R. (2001). *Managing Aggression*. London and New York: Routledge.

Brayden, R.M., Deitrich-MacLean, G., Dietrich, M.S., Sherrod, K.B., and Altemeier, W.A. (1995). Evidence for specific effects of childhood sexual abuse on mental well-being and physical self-esteem. *Child Abuse and Neglect*, 19(10), 1255–62.

Brennan, F. (2003). *Tampering with Asylum. A Universal Humanitarian Problem*. Brisbane: University of Queensland Press.

Brewer, P. (2002). *Has Identity Politics Shifted Feminism to the Right*. Paper presented at the Jubilee Conference of the Australasian Political Studies Association, Canberra.

Bridget, J. and Lucille, S. (1996). Lesbian Youth Support Information Services (LYSIS); Developing a distance support agency for young lesbians. *Journal of Community and Applied Social Psychology*, 6(5), 355–64.

Broverman, I., Broverman, D.M., Clarkson, I.E., Rosenkrantz, P.S. and Vogel, S.R. (1970). Sex role stereotypes and clinical judgements of mental health. *Journal of Consulting and Clinical Psychology*, 34, 1–7.

Brown, G.W. and Harris, T. (1978). *Social Origins of Depression*. London: Tavistock Publications.

Brown, K., Puller, K. and Bradley, L. (2006, July 2006). *Transition from Domestic Violence to Sustainable Employment in an Era of WorkChoices*. Paper presented at the National conference on women's Industrial Relations: Our Work ... Our Lives, Griffith University, Brisbane.

Brown, L.S. (1996). Preventing heterosexism and bias in psychotherapy and counseling. In E.D. Rothblum and L.A. Bond (eds), *Preventing Heterosexism and Homophobia*. London: Sage.

Brown, R.M. (1976). *A Plain Brown Rapper*. Oakland, CA: Dianna Press.

Brownmiller, S. (1975). *Against Our Will: Men, Women and Rape*. New York: Simon & Schuster.

Brunetto, Y. and Farr-Wharton, R. (2005). The role of management post-NPM in the implementation of new policies affecting police officers' practices. *Policing – an International Journal of Police Strategies & Management*, 28(2), 221–41.

Bryson, V. (1999). *Feminist Debates, Issues of Theory and Practice*. New York: New York University Press.

Bryson, V. (2002). Recent feminisms: beyond dichotomies. *Contemporary Politics*, 8(3), 233–8.

Budd, T. (1999). *Violence at Work: Findings from the British Crime Survey*. London: Home Office.

Bunch, C. (1975). Not for lesbians only. *Quest, II*(2), 50–6.

Burdekin Report. (1993). *Human Rights and Mental Illness. Report of the National Inquiry into Rights of People with Mental Illness*. Canberra: Australian Government Printing.

Burgman, V. (2003). A Sorry Tale of Exclusion: The Howard Government versus Indigenous Australians 1996–2003. In D. Weiss (ed.), *Social Exclusion in Australia: An Approach to the Australian Case*. Frankfurt am Main: Peter Lang.

Burns, A., Burns, K. and Menzies, K. (1999). Strong state intervention: The stolen generations. In J. Bowes and A. Hayes (eds), *Children, Families and Communities: Contexts and Consequences*. Melbourne: Oxford University Press.

Burris, B. (1973). The Fourth World Manifesto. In A. Koedt, E. Levine and A. Rapone (eds), *Radical Feminism* (pp. 322–57). New York: Quadrangle.

Burstow, B. (2003). Toward a radical understanding of trauma and trauma work. *Violence Against Women, 9*(11), 1293–1317.

Burstow, B. (2004). 'Progressive psychotherapists and the psychiatric survivor movement'. *Journal of Humanistic Psychology, 44*(2), 141–54.

Burstow, B. and Weitz, D. (1988). Shrink Resistant: *The Struggle Against Psychiatry in Canada*. Vancouver: New Star Books.

Busfield, J. (1996). *Men, Women and Madness: Understanding Gender and Mental Disorder* London: Macmillan.

Butterworth, P. (2003). Multiple and severe disadvantage among lone mothers receiving income support. *Family Matters, 64*(Winter), 22–9.

Bytheway, B. (1995). *Ageism*. Buckingham and Philadelphia: Open University Press.

Cagatay, N., Grown, C. and Santiago, A. (1986). The Nairobi Women's Conference: toward a global feminism. *Feminist Studies, 12*(2), 401–12.

Caine, B. (1995). Women's studies, feminist traditions and the problem of history, Chapter 1. In B. Caine and R. Pringle (eds), *Transitions, New Australian Feminisms* (pp. 1–14). St Leonards: Allen and Unwin.

Calder, M., Harold, G. and Howarth, E. (2004). *Children Living with Domestic Violence. Towards a Framework for Assessment and Intervention*. Dorset: Russell House Publishing.

Calhoun, C. (ed.). (2002). *Dictionary of Social Sciences*. New York: Oxford University Press.

Calma, T. (2006). *Ending Family Violence and Abuse in Aboriginal and Torres Strait Islander Communities – Key Issues: An overview paper of research and findings by the Human Rights and Equal Opportunity Commission, 2001–2006*: Human Rights and Equal Opportunity Commission.

Cammiss, S. (2006). The management of domestic violence cases in the mode of trial hearing: Prosecutorial control and marginalizing victims. *British Journal of Criminology, 46*(4), 704–718.

Campaign, E.V.A.W. (2006). Why End Violence Against Women? Retrieved 13 December 2007, from http://www.endviolenceagainstwomen.org.uk/home.asp#

Campbell, H. and Phillips, E. (1997). Masculine hegemony and leisure sites in rural New Zealand and Australia. In P. Share (ed.), *Communication and Culture in Rural Areas* (Vol. Key Papers Series 4). Wagga Wagga: Centre for Rural Social Research.

Campbell, J., Rose, L., Kub, J. and Nedd, D. (1998). Voices of strength and resistance: A contextual and longitudinal analysis of women's responses to battering. *Journal of Interpersonal Violence, 13*(6), 743–62.

Campbell, L. (1997). Family involvement in decision-making in child protection and care: Four types of case conferences. *Child and Family Social Work, 2*, 1–11.

Campbell, P. (2002). The services user/survivor movement. In C. Newnes, G. Holmes and C. Dunn (eds), *This is Madness*. Llangarron: PCCS Books.

Canadian Broadcasting Commission. (2004). Canada Accused of Ignoring Violence Against Aboriginal Women. *CBC TV News*. Toronto. (Accessed October 2006)

Carlson, B.E., McNutt, L.A., Choi, D.Y. and Rose, I.M. (2002). Intimate partner abuse and mental health. *Violence Against Women*, *8*(6), 720–45.

Carrigan, T., Connell, R. and Lee, J. (1987). Hard and heavy: Toward a new sociology of masculinity. In M. Kaufman (ed.), *Beyond Patriarchy: Essays by Men on Pleasure, Power and Change*. Toronto: Oxford.

Carrington, K. and Phillips, J. (2003). Domestic violence in Australia – an Overview of the Issues [electronic version]. Retrieved 25 September 2006, from http://www.aph.gov.au/library/intguide/ sP/Som_violence.htm.

Cashmore, J., Higgins, D., Bromfield, L. and Scott, D. (2006). Recent Australian child protection and out-of-home care research. What's been done – and what needs to be done? *Children Australia*, *31*(2), 4–11.

Cavanagh, K. (2003). Understanding women's responses to domestic violence. *Qualitative Social Work*, *2*(3), 229–49.

Cavanagh, K., Dobash, R. and Dobash, R. (2005). Men who murder children inside and outside the family. *British Journal of Social Work*, *35*, 667–88.

Cemlyn, S., and Briskman, L. (2003). Asylum, children's rights and social work. *Child and Family Social Work*, *8*, 163–78.

Chamberlin, J. (1978). *On Our Own: Patient-controlled Alternatives to the Mental Health system*. New York: Hawthorn Books.

Chamberlin, J. (1990). The ex-patients' movement: Where we've been and where we're going. *Journal of Mind and Behavior*, *11*(4), 323–8.

Chantler, K. (2006). Independence, dependency and interdependence: struggles and resistances of minoritized women within and on leaving violent relationships. *Feminist Review*, (82), 26–48.

Chappell, D. (2001). International trends in workplace violence: An overview. *Journal of Occupational Health and Safety, Australia and New Zealand*, *16*(5), 395–401.

Chappell, D. and Di Martino, V. (2000). *Violence at Work* (2nd edn). Geneva: International Labour Organization.

Chesler, P. (2005). *The Death of Feminism: What's Next in the Struggle for Women's Freedom?* New York: Palgrave Macmillan.

Choules, K. (2006). Globally privileged citizenship. *Race, Ethnicity and Education*, *9*(3), 275–93.

Christie, A. (2003). Unsettling the 'social' in social work: Responses to asylum seeking children in Ireland. *Child and Family Social Work*, *8*, 223–31.

Chung, D., Kennedy, R., O'Brien, B. and Wendt, S. (2000). *Home Safe Home: The Link between Domestic and Family Violence and Women's homelessness*. Canberra: Commonwealth Government.

Clark, V. (2006). Group work practice with Australian asylum seekers. *Australian Social Work*, *59*(4), 378–90.

Clarke, L. (2004). *The Time of the Therapeutic Communities*. London: Jessica Kingsley Publishers.

CLIT Collective. (1974). The agent within. In S. Hoagland and J. Penelope (eds), *For Lesbians Only. A Separatist Anthology* (pp. 371–9). London: Onlywoman Press.

Cocks, E. (1989). *An Introduction to Intellectual Disability in Australia*. Canberra: Australian Institute on Intellectual Disability.

Cohen, A. (1985). *The Symbolic Construction of Community*. London: Tavistock Publications.

Cohen, O. (2005). How do we recover? An analysis of psychiatric survivor oral histories. *Journal of Humanistic Psychology, 45*(3), 333–54.

Coker, D. (2000). Shifting power for battered women: Law, material resources, and poor women of colour. *University of California Law Review, 33*, 1009–55.

Coker, D. (2001). Crime control and feminist law reform in domestic violence law: A critical review. *Buffalo Criminal Law Review, 4*(2), 801–60.

Coker, D. (2004). Race, poverty, and the crime-centred response to domestic violence. *Violence Against Women, 10*(11), 1331–53.

Collins, L.H. (1998). Illustrating feminist theory: Power and psychopathology. *Psychology of Women Quarterly, 22*(1), 97–112.

Commission for Social Development. (2002a). *Abuse of Older Persons: Recognizing and Responding to Abuse of Older Persons in a Global Context*. New York: United Nations, Economic and Social Council.

Commission for Social Development. (2002b). *Research Agenda on Ageing for the 21st Century*. New York: United Nations.

Commonwealth of Australia. (2006). Criminal Code Amendment (Suicide Related Material Offences) Act 2005, *Criminal Code Act 1995*.

Connell, R.W. (1987). *Gender and Power: Society, the Person and Sexual Politics*. Sydney: Allen and Unwin.

Connell, R.W. (2000). *The Men and the Boys*. St Leonards: Allen and Unwin.

Connell, R.W. (2005). *Masculinities* (2nd edn). Berkeley: University of California Press.

Connolly, M., Crichton-Hill, Y. and Ward, T. (2006). *Culture and Child Protection*. London: Jessica Kingsley Publishers.

Conrad, D. and Kellar-Guenther, Y. (2006). Compassion fatigue, burnout and compassion satisfaction among Colarado child protection workers. *Child Abuse & Neglect, 30*(10), 1071–80.

Cook, J. and Watt, S. (1992). Racism, women and poverty. In C. Glendinning and J. Millar (eds), *Women and Poverty in Britain: the 1990s*. London: Harvester.

Cooper, D. (1993). *Child Abuse Revisited. Children, Society and Social Work*. Buckingham: Open University Press.

Coorey, L. (1990). Domestic Violence in Rural Areas. In M. Alston (ed.), *Key Papers: Number 1 – Rural Women* (pp. 37–53). Wagga Wagga: Centre for Rural Social Research.

Corby, B. (2000). *Child Abuse. Towards a Knowledge Base* (2nd edn). Buckingham: Open University Press.

Correa-Velez, I., Gifford, S. and Bice, S. (2005). Australian health policy on access to medical care for refugees and asylum seekers. *Australian and New Zealand Health Policy*.

Costello, M., Chung, D. and Carson, E. (2005). Exploring alternative pathways out of poverty: Making connections between domestic violence and employment practices. *Australian Journal of Social Issues, 40*(2), 253–67.

Cox, T. and Griffith, A. (1994). *Manual on Occupational Stress in Nursing*. Geneva: International Labour Organization.

Cree, V. and Wallace, S. (2005). Risk and protection. In R. Adams, L. Dominelli and M. Payne (eds), *Social Work Futures: Crossing Boundaries Transforming practice* (pp. 115–27). Basingstoke: Palgrave Macmillan.

Crenshaw, K.W. (1991). Mapping the margins: Intersectionality, identity politics and violence against women of color. *Stanford Law Review, 43*, 1241–99.

Cretney, A. and Davis, G. (1997). Prosecuting domestic assault: Victims failing courts, or courts failing victims? *The Howard Journal, 36*(2), 146–57.

Dalgleish, L. (2004). *Steps to a Decision Making Ecology for Child Protective Services: A Multi-National Research Perspective.* Paper presented at the 15th International Conference on Child Abuse and Neglect.

Dalley, G. (1993). The principles of collective care. In J. Bornat, C. Pereira, D. Pilgrim and E. Williams (eds), *Community Care: A Reader.* Basingstoke: Macmillan.

Daly, M. (1973). *Beyond God the Father: Towards a Philosophy of Women's Liberation.* Boston: Beacon Press.

Daly, M. (1978). *Gyn/ecology: The Metaethics of Radical Feminism.* Boston: Beacon Press.

Daniel, B., Featherstone, B., Hooper, C. and Scourfield, J. (2005). Why gender matters to *Every Child Matters. British Journal of Social Work, 35,* 1343–55.

Daniel, B., Wassell, S. and Gilligan, R. (1999). *Child Development for Child Care and Protection Workers.* London: Jessica Kingsley Publishers.

Das Gupta, S. (2003). Safety and justice for all: Examining the relationship between the women's anti-domestic violence movement and the legal system. Retrieved 7 December 2006, from http:// www.ms.foundation.org/user-assets/PDF/Program/safety_justice.pdf

Davidson, N., Skull, S., Chaney, G., Frydenberg, A., Issaacs, D., Kelly, P., et al. (2004). Comprehensive health assessment for newly arrived refugee children in Australia. *Journal of Paediatrics and Child Health, 40*(9–10), 562–8.

Davies, J., Lyon, E. and Monti-Catania, D. (1998). *Safety Planning with Battered Women: Complex Lives/Difficult Choices.* Thousand Oaks, CA: Sage.

Davies, K. (1993). On the movement. In J. Swain, V. Finkelstein, S. French and M. Oliver (eds), *Disabling Barriers and Enabling Environments.* London: Sage.

Davis, K. (1993) On the Movement. In J. Swain, V. Finkelstein, S. French and M. Oliver (eds), *Disabling Barriers – Enabling Environments.* London: Sage.

Day Sclater, B. and Yates, C. (1999). The psych-politics of post-divorce parenting. In A. Bainham, S. Day Sclater and M. Richards (eds), *What is a Parent? A Socio-Legal Analysis.* Oxford: Hart Publishing.

D'Cruz, H. (2004). *Constructing Meanings and Identities in Child Protection Practice.* Croyden: Tertiary Press.

De Albornoz, S. (2006). Failure to tackle refugees' health needs increase risk of exclusion. *British Medical Journal, 333,* 517.

De Beauvoir, S. (1974). *The Second Sex.* New York: Vantage.

De Leo, D. and Heller, T. (2004). Who are the kids who self-harm? An Australian self-report school survey. *Medical Journal of Australia, 181*(3), 140–4.

De Maria, W. (1996). The welfare whistleblower: In praise of troublesome people. *Australian Social Work, 49*(3), 15–24.

De Maria, W. and Jan, C. (1994). *Wounded Workers, Queensland Whistleblower Study.* Brisbane: Department of Social Work and Social Policy, University of Queensland.

De Panfallis, D. (2006). Compassion fatigue, burnout, and compassion satisfaction: Implications for retention of workers. *Child Abuse & Neglect, 30*(10), 1067–70.

Dean, H. (2003). Re-conceptualising Welfare-To-Work for people with multiple problems and needs. *Journal of Social Policy, 32*(3), 441–59.

Dekel, R. and Peled, E. (2000). Staff burnout in Israeli battered women's shelters. *Journal of Social Service Research, 26*(3), 65–76.

Dempsey, K. (1992a). *Smalltown. A Study of Social Inequality, Cohesion and Belonging.* Oxford: Oxford University Press.

Dempsey, K. (2002b). Community: Its Character and Meaning. In P. Beilharz and T. Hogan (eds), *Social Self, Global Culture: An Introduction to Sociological Ideas* (2nd edn). Melbourne: Oxford University Press.

Department of Economic and Social Affairs. (2004). *World Population Prospects: The 2004 Revision. Analytical Report.* Geneva: United Nations.

Department of Economic and Social Affairs. (2005). *Report on the World Social Situation. The Inequality Predicament* Geneva: United Nations.

Department of Health. (1999). *National Service Framework for Mental Health: Modern Standards and Service Models.* London: The Stationery Office.

Department of Health. (2000). *No Secrets: Guidance on Developing Multi-agency Policies and Procedures to Protect Vulnerable Adults from Abuse.* London: Home Office.

Department of Health. (2003b). *Delivering Race Equality: A Framework for Action.* London: The Stationery Office.

Department of Health. (2003a). *Inside/Outside: Improving Mental Health Services for Black and Minority Ethnic Communities in England.* London: National Institute for Mental Health in England.

Department of Health. (2004). *Protection of Vulnerable Adults (POVA) Scheme in England and Wales for Care Homes and Domiciliary Agencies.* London Home Office.

Department of Health (NSW). (2006). *A Statewide Approach to Measuring and Responding to Consumer Perceptions and Experiences of Adult Mental Health Services: A Report on Stage One of the Development of the MH-CoPES Framework and Questionnaires.* Sydney: NSW Department of Health.

Di Bartolo, L. (2001). The geography of reported domestic violence in Brisbane: a social justice perspective. *Australian Geographer, 32*(3), 321–41.

Di Martino, V. and Musri, M. (2001). *Guidance for the Prevention of Stress and Violence in the Workplace.* Department of Occupational Safety and Health, Ministry of Human Resources, Malaysia.

Diekstra, R. (1987). Renee or the complex psychodynamics of adolescent suicide. In R. Diekstra and K. Hawton (eds), *Suicide in Adolescence.* Dordrecht: Martinus Nijhoff.

Dobash, R., Dobash, R., Cavanagh, K. and Lewis, R. (2000). *Changing Violent Men.* London: Sage.

Dobash, R.E. and Dobash, R.P. (1992). *Women, Violence and Social Change.* London and New York: Routledge.

Dobash, R.E. and Dobash, R.P. (1998). Violent men and violent contexts. In R.E. Dobash and R.P. Dobash (eds), *Rethinking Violence Against Women.* Thousand Oaks, CA: Sage.

Dobash, R.P., Dobash, R.E., Wilson, M. and Daly, M. (1992). The myth of sexual symmetry in marital violence. *Social Problems, 39*(1), 71–91.

Douglas, H. and Godden, L. (2003). The decriminalisation of domestic violence: examining the interaction between the criminal law and domestic violence. *Criminal Law Journal, 27*(1), 32–43.

Dowd, N.E. (2006). Introduction. In N.E. Dowd, D.G. Singer and R.F. Wilson (eds), *Handbook of Children, Culture and Violence.* London: Sage.

Duffy, E. (1995). Horizontal violence: A conundrum for nursing. *Royal College of Nursing, Australia Collegian, 2*(2), 5–17.

Duggan, M., Cooper, A. and Foster, J. (2002). Modernising the social model in mental health: A discussion paper [Electronic Version] from www.topss.org.uk/uk_eng.

Durkheim, E. (1952). *Suicide: A Study in Sociology.* London: Routledge.

Durr, P. and Pona, I. (2003) Dreams, Struggles and Survivors – Messages from Young Refugees. In The Children's Society (2004), *Submission of the Children's Society, The*

Joint Committee on Human Rights Inquiry into the UN Committee on the Elimination of *Racial Discrimination's Concluding Observations on the UK's Compliance with the Convention on the Elimination of All Forms of Racial Descrimination*. Retrieved 12 February 2007, from http://www.the-childrens-society.org.uk/media/pdf/submissionto JCHRonracialdiscrinationNov04.pdf

Durr, P. and Pona, I. (2004). Dreams, struggles and survivors – Messages from young refugees. *The Children's Society*.

Dutton, D. (1994). Patriarchy and wife assault: The ecological fallacy. *Violence and Victims*, 9, 167–82.

Dutton, M.A. (1996). Battered women's strategic response to violence: The role of context. In J.L. Edleson and Z.C. Eisikovits (eds), *Future Interventions with Battered Women and their Families*. Thousand Oaks, CA: Sage.

Dutton, M.A. and Goodman, L.A. (2005). Coercion in intimate partner violence: Toward a new conceptualization. *Sex Roles*, 52(11–12), 743–56.

Dworkin, A. (1981). *Pornography: Men Possessing Women*. New York: Perigree Books.

Eaton, M. (1994). Abuse by any other name: Feminism, difference and intralesbian violence. In M.A. Fineman and R. Mykitiuk (eds), *The Public Nature of Private Violence* (pp. 195–224). New York: Routledge.

Echols, A. (1989). *Daring to be Bad. Radical Feminism in America, 1967–1975*. Minneapolis: University of Minnesota Press.

Economic and Social Research Council. (2006). Health and well-being of working age people, ESRC Seminar Series, Mapping the public policy landscape: Published jointly by the ESRC, the Department of Health, the Department for Work and Pensions and the Health and Safety Executive. UK.

Edleson, J. (1999). Children witnessing of adult domestic violence. *Journal of Interpersonal Violence*, 14, 839–70.

Edwards, A. (1987). Male violence in feminist theory: An analysis of the changing conceptions of sex/gender violence and male domination. In J. Hanmer and M. Maynard (eds), *Women, Violence and Social Control* (pp. 13–29). London: Macmillan.

Edwards, R. (2004a). *Staying Home Leaving Violence: Promoting Choices for Women Leaving Abusive Partners*. Sydney: Australian Domestic and Family Violence Clearinghouse. Available online: http://www.austdvclearinghouse.unsw/edu.au/topics.htm [accessed 20 January 2007].

Edwards, R. (2004b). *Violence excluded: a study into exclusion orders in South East Sydney*. Sydney: Attorney General's Department of NSW.

Eisenbruch, M. (1991). From post-traumatic stress disorder to cultural bereavement: Diagnosis of Southeast Asian refugees. *Social Science and Medicine*, 33(6), 673–680.

Elder, B. (1998). *Blood on the Wattle: Massacres and Maltreatment of Aboriginal Australians since 1788*: New Holland.

Eley, S. (2005). Changing practices: The specialised domestic violence court process. *The Howard Journal*, 44(2), 113–24.

English, D., Hollibaugh, A. and Rubin, G. (1982). Talking sex: A conversation on sexuality and feminism. *Socialist Review*, 17(3 & 4), 9–34.

Epstein, D. (1999). Effective intervention in domestic violence cases: Rethinking the roles of prosecutors, judges, and the court system. *Yale Journal of Law and Feminism*, 11(3), 3–50.

Epstein, D., Bell, M. and Goodman, L.A. (2003). Transforming aggressive prosecution policies: Prioritizing victims' long-term safety in the prosecution of domestic violence cases. *American University Journal of Gender Social Policy & the Law*, 11(2), 465–98.

Erez, E. and Belknap, J. (1998). In their own words: Battered women's assessment of the criminal processing system's response. *Violence and Victims, 13*(3), 251–68.

Erikson, K. (1976). *Everything in its Path*. New York: Simon and Schuster.

Erikson, K. (1994). *A New Species of Trouble: The Human Experience of Modern Disaster*. New York: Norton.

Eriksson, E. and Hester, M. (2001). Violent men as good-enough fathers? A look at England and Sweden. *Violence Against Women, 7*(7), 779–98.

Esienbruch, M. (1991). From post-traumatic stress disorder to cultural bereavement: Diagnosis of south east Asian refugees. *Social Science Medical, 33*(6), 673–80.

Estes, C. (1979). *The Aging Enterprise*. San Fanscisco: Jossey-Bass Publishers.

European Parliament. (2005). Turning the spotlight on violence against women: Background information OnlineAccessed 15.6.2006 [Electronic Version]. Retrieved 15 June 2006, from http://www.europarl.eu.int/omk/sipad3?

Evans, S. (2005). Beyond gender: Class, poverty and domestic violence. *Australian Social Work, 58*(1), 36–43.

Farberow, N. (1994). Preparatory and prior suicidal behavior factors. In E. Shneidman, N. Farberow and R. Litman (eds), *The Psychology of Suicide: A Clinician's Guide to Evaluation and Treatment*. New Jersey: Jason Aronson Inc.

Farberow, N., Heilig, S. and Litman, R. (1994). Evaluation and management of suicidal persons. In E. Shneidman, N. Farberow and R. Litman (eds), *The Psychology of Suicide: A Clinician's Guide to Evaluation and Treatment*. New Jersey: Jason Aronson Inc.

Fawcett, B. and Featherstone, B. (1998). Quality assurance and evaluation in social work in a modern era. In J. Carter (ed.), *Postmodernity and the Fragmentation of Welfare. A Contemporary Social Policy* (pp. 67–87). London: Routledge.

Fawcett, B. (2000). *Feminist Perspectives on Disability*. New York: Prentice Hall/Pearson.

Fawcett, B., Featherstone, B., and Goddard, J. (2004). *Contemporary Child Care Policy and Practice*. Basingstoke: Palgrave Macmillan.

Fawcett, B. and Karban, K. (2005). *Contemporary Mental Health: Theory, Policy and Practice*. London: Routledge.

Fazel, M., and Silove, D. (2006). Detention of refugees, editorial. *British Medical Journal, 332*, 251–52.

Fazel, M., and Stein, A. (2002). The mental health of refugee children. *Archives of Disease in Childhood, 87*, 366–70.

Featherstone, B. (2004). *Family Life and Family Support: A Feminist Analysis*. New York and Basingstoke: Palgrave Macmillan.

Featherstone, B. and Peckover, S. (2007). Letting them get away with it: Fathers, domestic violence and child welfare. *Journal of Critical Social Policy, 27*(2): 181–203.

Ferguson, H. (2003). Welfare, social exclusion and reflexivity: The case of child and woman protection *Journal of Social Policy, 32*(2), 119–26.

Fernando, S., Ndegwa, D. and Wilson, M. (1998). *Forensic Psychiatry, Race and Culture*. London: Routledge.

Ferraro, K. and Pope, L. (1993). Irreconcilable differences: Battered women, police, and the law. In N.Z. Hilton (ed.), *Legal Responses to Wife Assault: Current Trends and Evaluation* (pp. 96–123). Newbury Park, CA: Sage.

Ferreira, M. (2004). Elder abuse in Africa: What policy and legal provision are there to address the violence? *Journal of Elder Abuse & Neglect, 16*(2), 17–32.

Figley, C. (1985). *Trauma and its Wake: The Study Treatment of Post-traumatic Stress Disorder* New York: Brunner/Mazel.

Fineman, M.A. and Mykitiuk, R. (eds). (1994). *The Public Nature of Private Violence: The Discovery of Domestic Abuse*. New York: Routledge.

Finkelstein, V. (1991). Disability: an administrative challenge? In M. Oliver (ed.), *Social Work, Disabled People and Disabling Environments*. London: Jessica Kingsley Publishers.

Firestone, S. (1970). *The Dialectic of Sex*. New York: Bantam Books.

Fitzgerald, J. and Weatherburn, D. (2002). Aboriginal victimisation and offending: the picture from police records. *Aboriginal and Islander Health Worker Journal, 26*(4), 26–8.

Fleury-Steiner, R.E., Bybee, D., Sullivan, C.M., Belknap, J., and Melton, H.C. (2006). Contextual factors impacting battered women's intentions to reuse the criminal legal system. *Journal of Community Psychology, 34*(3), 327–42.

Fook, J. (2002). *Social Work: Critical Theory and Practice*. London: Sage.

Forbat, L. (2004). The care and abuse of minoritized ethnic groups: the role of statutory services. *Critical Social Policy, 24*(3), 312–31.

Ford, D.A. and Regoli, M.J. (1993). The criminal prosecution of wife assaulters: Process, problems and effects. In N.Z. Hilton (ed.), *Legal Responses to Wife Assault: Current Trends and Evaluation* (pp. 127–64). Newbury Park, CA: Sage.

Foucault, M. (1979). *Discipline and Punish*. Harmondsworth: Penguin.

Foucault, M. (1980). Michel Foucault. In C. Gordon (ed.), *Power/Knowledge: Selected Interviews and Other Writings*. Hemel Hempstead: Harvester Wheatsheaf.

Foucault, M. (1986). *The History of Sexuality. Volume Two: The Use of Pleasure*. Harmondsworth: Viking.

Fox, C. and Hawton, K. (2004). *Deliberate Self-Harm in Adolescence*. London: Jessica Kingsley Publishers.

Fraidlin, N. and Rabin, B. (2006). Social workers confront terrorist victims: the interventions and the difficulties. *Social Work in Health Care, 43*(2/3), 115–31.

Frank, R. (2003). When bad things happen in good places: Pastoralism in big-city newspaper coverage of small-town violence. *Rural Sociology, 68*(2), 207.

Frankl, V. (1963). *Man's Search for Meaning*. Boston: Pocket Books.

Fraser, H. (2002). *Narrating Love and Abuse in Social Work: A Critical Postmodern Feminist Perspective*. Unpublished PhD Thesis, University of Melbourne, Melbourne.

Fraser, K. (2003). *Domestic Violence and Women's Physical Health*. Sydney: Australian Domestic and Family Violence Clearinghouse.

Fraser, M., Richman, J. and Galinsky, M. (1999). Risk, protection and resilience: Toward a conceptual framework for social work practice. *Social Work Research, 23*(3), 131–43.

Fraser, N. and Nicholson, L. (1993). Social Criticism Without Philosophy: An Encounter Between Feminism and Postmodernism. In M Docherty (ed.), *Postmodernism: A Reader*. Hemel Hempstead: Harvester Wheatsheaf.

Freeman, D.W. and Fallot, R.D. (1997). Trauma and trauma recovery for dually diagnosed male survivors. In M. Harris and C.L. Landis (eds), *Sexual Abuse in the Lives of Women Diagnosed with Serious Mental Illness*. London: Harwood Academic.

French, H. (2007, 1 April). China faces a looming crisis as its workers near old age. *The New York Times* (p. 1). New York.

Frye, M. (1983). *The Politics of Reality: Essays in Feminist Theory*. Trumansburg, NY: Crossing Press.

Gabarino, J. (1999) *Lost Boys: Why Our Sons Turn Violent and How We Can Save Them*. New York: Free Press.

Gailiene, D. (2004). Suicide in Lithuania during the years of 1990 and 2002. *Archives of Suicide Research, 8*, 389–95.

Galtung, J. and Hoivik, T. (1971). Structural and direct violence: A note on operational-ization. *Journal of Peace Research*, *8*(1), 73.

Garbarino, J. (1981). An ecological approach to child maltreatment. In L. Pelton (ed.), *The Social Contect of Child Abuse and Neglect* New York: Human Services Press.

Garbarino, J. (1992). *Children and Families in the Social Environment* (2nd edn). New York: Aldine de Gruyter.

Garner, J.H. and Maxwell, C.D. (2000). What are the lessons of the police arrest studies? In S.K. Ward and D. Finkelhor (eds), *Program Evaluation and Family Violence Research*. New York: The Haworth Maltreatment and Trauma Press.

Genovese, A. (2000). The politics of naming: '70s feminisms, genealogy and 'domestic Violence'. In R. Walker, K. Brass and J. Byron (eds), *Anatomies of Violence: An Interdisciplinary Investigation*. (pp. 115–128). Sydney: Postgraduate Arts Research Centre and the Research Institute for Humanities and Social Sciences, University of Sydney.

Gershoff, E. (2002). Corporal punishment by parents and associated child behaviours and experiences: a meta-analysis and theoretical review. *Psychological Bulletin*, *128*, 539–79.

Gillingham, P. (2006). Risk assessment in child protection: Problem rather than solution? *Australian Social Work*, *59*(1), 86–98.

Girshick, L.B. (2002). *Woman-to-Woman Sexual Violence*. Boston: Northeastern University Press.

Goddard, C., and Carew, R. (1993). *Responding to Children*. Melbourne: Longman Cheshire.

Goffman, E. (1961). *Asylums*. London and Chicago: Allen Lane.

Goffman, E. (1963). *Stigma: Notes on the Management of Spoiled Identity*. Englewood Cliffs, NJ: Prentice-Hall.

Goodman, L., Bennett, L. and Dutton, M.A. (1999). Obstacles to victims' cooperation with the criminal prosecution of their abusers: The role of social support. *Violence and Victims*, *14*(4), 427–44.

Goodman, L. and Epstein, D. (2005). Refocusing on women: A new direction for policy and research on intimate partner violence. *Journal of Interpersonal Violence*, *20*(4), 479–87.

Goodwin, S. (2005). Community and social inclusion. In P. Smyth, T. Reddel and A. Jones (eds), *Community and Local Governance in Australia* (pp. 94–107). Sydney: UNSW Press.

Goonesekere, S. (ed.). (2004). *Violence, Law and Women's Rights in South Asia*. New Delhi: Sage and UNIFEM South Asia Regional Office.

Gordon, S., Hallahan, K. and Henry, D. (2002). *Putting the Picture Together: Inquiry into Response by Government Agencies to Complaints of Family Violence and Child Abuse in Aboriginal Communities*. Perth: State Law Publisher, Western Australia.

Gould Davis, E. (1972). *The First Sex*. New York: Penguin.

Griffin, S. (1979). *Rape: The Power of Consciousness*. San Francisco: Harper and Rowe.

Gutierree, L.M., Parsons, R.J. and Cox, E.O. (1998). *Empowerment in Social Work Practice*. CA: Brooks/Cole.

Gutter Dyke Collective. (1988). This is the year to stamp out the 'Y'. In S. Hoagland and J. Penelope (eds), *For Lesbians Only* (pp. 338–9). London: Onlywomen Press.

Hague, G. and Mallos, E. (1993). *Domestic Violence: Action for Change*. Cheltenham: New Clarion Press.

Hanmer, J. (1978). Violence and the social control of women. In G. Littlejohn, C. Smart and J. Hanmer (eds), *Power and the State* (pp. 217–38). London: Croom Helm.

Hanmer, J. and Itzin, C. (2000). Introduction: Prevention, provision and protection. In J. Hanmer and C. Itzin (eds), *Home Truths About Domestic Violence: Feminist Influences on Policy and Practice: A Reader* (pp. 1–6). London: Routledge.

Hanna, C. (1996). No right to choose: Mandated victim participation in domestic violence prosecutions. *Harvard Law Review, 109*(8), 1849–1910.

Hanna, C. (1998). The paradox of hope: The crime and punishment of domestic violence. *William and Mary Law Review, 39*(5), 1505–84.

Hannam, J. (2007). *Feminism.* Harlow: Pearson Education.

Harbison, J. and Morrow, M. (1998). Re-examining the social construction of 'elder abuse and neglect': A Canadian perspective. *Ageing and Society, 18*, 691–711.

Hardiman, E.R. (2004). 'Networks of caring: a qualitative study of social support in consumer-run mental health agencies'. *Qualitative Social Work, 3*(4), 431–48.

Harding, C.M., and Zahniser, J.H. (1994). Empirical correction of seven myths about schizophrenia with implications for treatment. A*cta Psychiatrica Scan Suppl, 384*, 140–6.

Harne, L. (2004). Childcare violence and fathering – are violent fathers who look after their children likely to be less abusive? In R. Klein and B. Wallner (eds), *Gender, Conflict and Violence.* Vienna: Studien-Verlag.

Harris, M. and Telfer, B. (2001). The health needs of asylum seekers living in the community. *Medical Journal of Australia, 175*, 589–92.

Harrison, G.K.H., Craig, T., Laska, E., Siegel, C., Wanderling, J., et al. (2001). Recovery from psychotic illness: A 15- and 25-year international follow-up study. *The British Journal of Psychiatry, 178*, 506–17.

Harrold, K. (1987). *Theoretical Approaches to the Etiology of Child Maltreatment.* Brisbane: Research and Evaluation Branch Department of Children's Services.

Hart, L., Larson, E. and Lishner, D. (2005). Rural definitions in health policy and research. *American Journal of Public Health, 95*(7), 1149–55.

Harwin, N. (2006). Putting a stop to domestic violence in the United Kingdom. *Violence Against Women, 12*(6), 556–7.

Hatfield, A.B. and Lefley, H.P. (1993). *Surviving Mental Illness.* New York: The Guilford Press.

Healthcare Commission. (2005). The 'Count Me In' Mental Health and Ethnicity Census. London: The Healthcare Commission.

Hearn, J. (1992). *Men in the Public Eye: The Construction and Destruction of Public Men and Public Patriarchies.* London: Routledge.

Hearn, J. (1996). Men's violence to known women: Historical, everyday and theoretical constructions by men. In B. Fawcett, B. Featherstone, J. Hearn and C. Tofts (eds), *Violence and Gender Relations: Theories and Interventions.* London: Sage.

Hearn, J. (1998). Men will be men: The ambiguity of men's support for men who have been violent to known women. In J. Popay, J. Hearn and J. Edwards (eds), *Men, Gender Divisions and Welfare.* London: Routledge.

Hearn, J. and McKie, L. (forthcoming). Gendered policy and policy on gender: the case of 'domestic violence', *Policy and Politics.*

Hearn, J. and Whitehead, A. (2006). Collateral damage: Men's 'domestic' violence to women seen through men's relations with men. *Journal of Community and Criminal Justice, 53*(1), 55–74.

Hegarty, M. (2004). *Mind the Gap.* Sydney: NSW Department of Community Services.

Heise, L. (1998). Violence against women. An integrated ecological framework. *Violence against Women, 4*(3), 262–90.

Heise, L., Ellsberg, M.C. and Gottmoeller, M. (2002). A global overview of gender-based violence. *International Journal of Gynecology and Obstetrics, 78 Suppl. 1*, S5–S14.

Herek, G.M. and Berril, K.T. (1990). Anti-gay violence and mental health: Setting an agenda for research. *Special Issue: Violence against lesbians and gay men: Issues for research, practice, and policy. Journal of Interpersonal Violence*, 5(3), 414–23.

Herman, J.L. (1992). *Trauma and Recovery: The Aftermath of Violence-from Domestic Abuse to Political Terror*. New York: Basic Books.

Hester, M., Pearson, C. and Harwin, N. (2007). *Making an Impact: Children and Domestic Violence, A Reader*. London: Jessica Kingsley Publishers.

Hindin, M.J. (2003). Understanding women's attitudes towards wife beating in Zimbabwe. *Bulletin of the World Health Organization*, 81(7), 501–8.

Hitosugi, M., Nagai, T. and Tokudome, S. (2007). A voluntary effort to save the youth suicide via the Internet in Japan. *International Journal of Nursing Studies*, 44(1), 157.

HMSO. (1974). *Report of the Committee of Inquiry into South Ockendon Hospital*. London: HMSO.

Hodes, M. (2002). Implication for psychiatric services of chronic civilian strife: young refugees in the UK. *Advances in Psychiatric Treatment*, 8, 366–74.

Hoel, H., Sparks, K. and Cooper, C. (2001). *The Cost of Violence/Stress At Work and the Benefits of a Violence/Stress-Free Working Environment. Report commissioned by the International Labour Organization Geneva*: Institute of Science and Technology, University of Manchester.

Hoffman, T. (2006, 3–4 August). *Impediments to Staff Support: The Dr Death Case at Bundaberg Hospital*. Paper presented at the Crisis Intervention in a Changing World. Critical Incident Stress Management Foundation Australia. Fourth Conference, Melbourne, Victoria.

Holder, R. (2001). Domestic and family violence: criminal justice interventions, issues paper, No. 3. *Issue Paper*. Retrieved 4 September 2006, from http://www.austdvclearinghouse. unsw.edu.au/ PDF%20files/issuespaper3.pdf

Holder, R. (2004). Research for change: The ACT Family Violence Intervention Program experience. In E. Moore (ed.), *WOW, Wellbeing of Women conference proceedings: research and practice: Community of Scholars, Gender Woman and Social Policy* (pp. 10–17). Wagga Wagga, N.S.W.: Charles Sturt University.

Holland, S. (1995). Interaction in women's mental health and neigbourhood development. In S. Fernando (ed.), *Mental Health in a Multi-ethnic Society*. London: Routledge.

Home Office. (2006). *Lessons Learned from Domestic Violence Enforcement Campaigns in 2006*: Home Office, London.

Hood, M. (1998). The interplay between poverty, unemployment, family disruption and all types of child abuse. *Children Australia*, 23(2), 28–32.

hooks, b. (1981). *Ain't I a Woman: Black Women and Feminism*. Boston: South End Press.

hooks, b. (1984). *Feminist Theory: From Margin to Center*. Boston: South End Press.

hooks, b. (1991). *Yearning, Race, Gender and Cultural Politics*. London: Turnaround Press.

Hopton, J. (2006). The future of critical psychiatry. *Critical Social Policy*, 26(1), 57–73.

Hornosty, J. (1995). *Wife Abuse in Rural Regions – structural problems in leaving abusive relationships: a case study in Canada*. Paper presented at the With a Rural Focus Conference. Australian Sociological Association, Wagga Wagga.

Houghton, C. (2006). Listen Louder: Working with Children and Young People. In C. Humphreys and J. Stanley (eds), *Domestic Violence and Child Protection: Directions for Good Practice* (pp. 82–94). London: Jessica Kingsley Publishers.

Howie, G. and Tauchert, A. (2004). Feminist dissonance: The logic of late feminism. In S. Gillis, G. Howie and R. Munford (eds), *Third Wave Feminism A critical Exploration* (pp. 37–48). New York: Palgrave Macmillan.

Hoyle, C. and Sanders, A. (2000). Police response to domestic violence: from victim choice to victim empowerment. *British Journal of Criminology, 40*, 14–36.

HREOC. (1997). *Bringing Them Home. Report of the National Inquiry into the Separation of Aboriginal and Torres Strait Islander Children from their Families.* Canberra: Commonwealth of Australia.

Hudson, M. (1999). Psychiatric hospitals and patients' councils. In C. Newnes, G. Holmes and C. Dunn (eds), *This is Madness: A Critical Look at Psychiatry and the Future of the Mental Health Services.* Ross-on-Wye: PCCS Books.

Hughes, H.M., Humphrey, N.N., and Weaver, T.L. (2005). Advances in violence and trauma: Toward comprehensive ecological models. *Journal of Interpersonal Violence, 20*(1), 31–8.

Hulme, P. (1996). Everybody means something: Collaborative conversations. *Changes – Sheffield, 14*(1), 67–72.

Human Rights and Equal Opportunity Commission. (1997). *Bringing Them Home: Report of the National Inquiry into the Separation of Aboriginal and Torres Strait Islander Children from their Families.* Sydney: Human Rights and Equal Opportunity Commission.

Humphreys, C. (1993). *The Referral of Families Associated with Child Sexual Assault.* Sydney: New South Wales, Department of Community Services.

Humphreys, C. (2006). Relevant evidence for practice. In C. Humphreys and N. Stanley (eds), *Domestic Violence and Child Protection* (pp. 19–35). London: Jessica Kingsley Publishers.

Humphreys, C. (2007). A health inequalities perspective on violence against women. *Health and Social Care in the Community, 15*(2), 120–7.

Humphreys, C., and Joseph, S. (2004). Domestic violence and the politics of trauma. *Women's Studies International Forum, 27*(5/6), 559–70.

Humphreys, C., Regan, L., River, D. and Thiara, R. (2005). Domestic violence and sub-stance abuse: Tackling complexity. *British Journal of Social Work, 35*, 1303–20.

Humphreys, C., and Stanley, N. (2006). Introduction. In C. Humphreys and N. Stanley (eds), *Domestic Violence and Child Protection.* London: Jessica Kingsley Publishers.

Humphreys, C. and Thiara, R. (2003). Mental health and domestic violence: 'I call it symptoms of abuse'. *British Journal of Social Work, 33*, 209–26.

Hung Suet Lin, S. (2006, 13 October). *Violence in Marriage – Immigrant Women Tell Their Stories.* Paper presented at the Symposium on Domestic Violence – Welfare of Children and Families, Hong Kong Baptist University.

Hunter, R. (2002). Border protection in law's empire: Feminist explorations of access to justice. *Griffith University Professorial Lecture.* Retrieved 15 October 2006, from http://www.gu.edu. au/ins/collections/proflects/hunter02.pdf

Hunter, R. (2005). Styles of judging: how magistrates deal with applications for interven-tion orders. *Alternative Law Journal, 30*(5), 231–46.

Hutchinson, G.S. and Weeks, W. (2004). Living conditions of women who experience vio-lence from their partners: Norway and Australia comparisons. *Australian Journal of Social Issues, 39*(4), 393–407.

Ife, J. (1997). *Rethinking Social Work: Towards Critical Practice.* South Melbourne: Longman.

Iriwn, J., Laing, L. and Napier, L. (2006, 28 August – 1 September). *Domestic Violence and Mental Health.* Paper presented at the 33rd International Congress of Schools of Social Work, Santiago, Chile.

Irwin, J. (2007, in press). Discounted Stories: Domestic violence and lesbians. *Qualitative Social Work.*

Irwin, J. (1999). *The Pink Ceiling is too Low:Workplace experiences of lesbians, gay men and transgender people. Report of a Collaborative Research Project undertaken by the Australian Centre for Lesbian and Gay Research and the NSW Gay and Lesbian Rights Lobby.* Sydney: Australian Centre for Lesbian and Gay Research, University of Sydney.

Irwin, J., Waugh, F. and Bonner, M. (2006). The inclusion of children and young people in research on domestic violence. *Communities, Families and Children Australia, 1*(1), 17–23.

Irwin, J., Waugh, F. and Wilkinson, M. (2000). *Domestic Violence and Child Protection: A research report.* Sydney: University of Sydney.

Irwin, L. and Waugh, F. (2001). *Unless They're Asked: Routine Screening for Domestic Violence in NSW Health: an evaluation report of the pilot project.* Sydney: NSW Health Department.

Island, D. and Letellier, P. (1991). *Men Who Beat the Men Who Love Them.* New York: Harrington Park Press.

Ismail, K. (1996). Planning services for black women. In K. Abel, M. Buszewics, S. Davison, S. Johnson and E. Staples (eds), *Planning Community Mental Health Services for Women.* London: Routledge.

Itzin, C. (2006). *Tackling the Health and Mental Health Effects of Domestic and Sexual Violence and Abuse.* London: Joint Department of Health and National Institute for Mental Health in England (NIMHE); Victims of Violence and Abuse Prevention Programme (VVAPP) Health and Mental Health, In Partnership with the Home Office.

Iverson, T. and Segal, M. (1990). *Child Abuse and Neglect.* New York: Garland Publishing.

Jacobson, N. and Curtis, L. (2000). Recovery as policy in mental health services: Strategies emerging from the States. *Psychiatric Rehabilitation Journal, 23*(4), 333–41.

James-Hanman, D. (2000). Enhancing multi-agency work. In J. Hanmer and C. Itzin (eds), *Home Truths About Domestic Violence: Feminist Influences on Policy and Practice: A Reader* (pp. 269–86). London: Routledge.

Jan, L.F. (1998). Social capital and communities of place. *Rural Sociology, 63*(4), 481.

Jategaonkar, N., Greaves, L., Poole, N., McCullough, L. and Chabot, C. (2005). 'Still out there': experiencing substance use and violence in rural British Columbia (analysis of abused women). *Canadian Woman Studies, 24.4*(Summer–Fall 2005), 136(136).

Jayaratne, S., Vinokur-Kaplan, D., Nagda, B. and Chess, W. (1996). A national study on violence and harrassment of social workers by clients. *Journal of Applied Social Sciences, 20*(1), 1–14.

Jejeebhoy, S. (1998). Wife-beating in rural India: a husband's right? *Economic and Political Weekly, 33*, 855–62.

Jianguo, G. and Li Qin. (2006, 13 October). *Domestic Violence in Rural China: An Exploration of Community Perspective.* Paper presented at the Symposium on domestic Violence – Welfare of Children and Families, Hong Kong Baptist University.

Joelsson, L. and Dahlin, K. (2005). The asylum seeking process: A breeding ground for apathy among certain children. A negative answer concerning the residence permit is often a triggering factor. *Lakartidningen, 102*(48), 3646–50.

Johnson, M. (1995). Patriarchal terrorism and common couple violence: two forms of violence against women. *Journal of Marriage and the Family, 57*, 283–94.

Johnston, J. (1974). *Lesbian Nation. The Feminist Solution.* New York: Touchstone.

Jones, A. (2001). Child asylum seekers and refugees. *Journal of Social Work, 1*(3), 253–71.

Kaplan, M. (1983). A woman's view of DSM-111. *American Psychologist, 38*, 788.

Kaschak, E. (ed.). (2001). *Intimate Betrayal: Domestic Violence in Lesbian Relationships.* New York: The Haworth Press Inc.

Katzen, H. (2000). It's a family matter, not a police matter: The enforcement of protection orders. *Australian Journal of Family Law*, *14*(2), 119–41.

Kaye/Kantrowitz, M. (1992). *The Issue of Power: Essays on Women, Jews, Violence and Resistance*. San Francisco: Aunt Lute Books.

Kaysen, S. (2000). *Girl, Interrupted*. London: Virago.

Keck, M. E. and Sikkink, K. (1998). *Activists Beyond Borders, Advocacy Networks in International Politics*. London: Cornell University Press.

Kelly, L. (1988). *Surviving Sexual Violence*. Minneapolis: University of Minnesota Press.

Kent, G. (2000). *State Violence Against Children. Committee on the Rights of the Child. Day of General Discussion*.

Keys Young. (2000). *Evaluation of ACT Interagency Family Violence Intervention Program: Final Report*. Canberra, ACT ACT Department of Justice and Community Safety.

Kim, J. and Motsei, M. (2002). 'Women enjoy punishment': attitudes and experiences of gender-based violence among PHC nurses in rural South Africa. *Social Science & Medicine*, *54*(8), 1243–54.

Kinnear, P. and Graycar, A. (1999). *Abuse of Older People: Crime or Family Dynamics?* Canberra: Australilan Institute of Criminology.

Kivimäki, K., Elovainio, M. and Vathera, J. (2000). Workplace bullying and sickness absence in hospital staff. *Occupational and Environmental Medicine*, *57*, 656–60.

Klein, E., Campbell, J., Soler, E. and Ghez, M. (1997). *Ending Domestic Violence: Changing Public Perceptions/Healing the Epidemic*. Thousand Oaks, CA: Sage.

Koenig, M.A., Lutalo, T., Zhao, F., Nalugoda, F., Wabwire-Mangen, F., Kiwanuka, N., et al. (2003). Domestic violence in rural Uganda: evidence from a community-based study. *Bulletin of the World Health Organization*, *81*(1), 53–60.

Kohli, R. (2006). The sound of silence: Listening to what unaccompaimed asylum seeking children say and do not say. *British Medical Journal*, *36*(5), 707–21.

Kurrle, S. (2004). Elder abuse. *Australian Family Physician*, *33*(10), 807–12.

Kvam, M. and Braathen, S. (2006). *Violence and Abuse Against Women with Disabilities in Malawi*. Oslo: SINTEF Health Research.

Kyeung, M. and Warnes, A. (2001). Care services for frail older people in South Korea. *Ageing and Society*, *21*(6), 701–7.

Laing, L. (2000). *Trends and Challenges in Australian Responses to Domestic Violence*. Sydney: University of New South Wales.

Laing, L. (2001). *Australian Studies of the Economic Costs of Domestic Violence*. Sydney: Australian Domestic and Family Violence Clearinghouse.

Laing, R.D. (1965). *The Divided Self*. Harmondsworth: Penguin.

Larbalestier, J. (1998). Identity and difference. In B. Caine (ed.), *Australian Feminism, A Companion* (pp. 148–58). Melbourne: Oxford University Press.

Leenaars, A., De Leo, D., Goldney, R., Gulbinat, W. and Wallace, M. (1998). Editorial. *Archives of Suicide Research*, *4*, 1–6.

Leifer, R. (2000). A critique of medical coercive psychiatry and an invitation to dialogue. *Ethical Human Science and Services*, *3*(3), 161–74.

Lempert, L.B. (1996). Women's strategies for survival: developing agency in abusive relationships. *Journal of Family Violence*, *11*(3), 269–89.

Lerner, M. (1991). *Surplus Powerlessness*. London: Humanities Press International.

Lester, D. and Yang, B. (2005). The base rate of suicide: Comment on 'A novel integrated knowledge explanation of factors leading to suicide'. *New Ideas in Psychology*, *23*(1), 49–51.

Lewis, B. (2006). *Moving Beyond Prozac, DSM, and the New Psychiatry: The Birth of Postpsychiatry*. Ann Arbor: The University of Michigan Press.

Lewis, R. (2004). Making justice work: Effective legal interventions for domestic violence. *British Journal of Criminology*, *44*(2), 204–24.

Lewis, R., Dobash, R.P., Dobash, R.E., and Cavanagh, K. (2000). Protection, prevention,
rehabilitation or justice? Women's use of the law to challenge domestic violence.
International Review of Victimology, *7*(1,2,3 special issue: Domestic Violence: Global
Responses), 179–205.

Leymann, H. (1990). Mobbing and psychological terror at workplaces. *Violence and
Victims*, *5*, 119–26.

Liddell, M., Donegan, T., Goddard, C. and Tucci , J. (2006). The state of child protection:
Australian child welfare and child protection developments 2005.

Lister, R. (2004). *Poverty*. Cambridge: Polity Press.

Litman, R. (1994). Responsibility and liability for suicide. In E. Shneidman, N. Farberow
and R. Litman (eds), *The Psychology of Suicide: A Clinician's Guide to Evaluation and
treatment*. New Jersey: Jason Aronson.

Lobel, K. (1986). Introduction. In K. Lobel (ed.), *Naming the Violence: Speaking Out
About Lesbian Battering* (pp. 1–8). Seattle WA: Seal Press.

Long, D.A. (2001). From support to self-sufficiency: how successful are programs in
advancing the financial independence and well-being of welfare recipients? *Education
and Program Planning*, *24*, 389–408.

Lucashenko, M. (1994). No other truth? Aboriginal women and Australian feminism.
Social Alternatives, *12*(4), 21–4.

Lutze, F.E., and Symons, M.L. (2003). The evolution of domestic violence policy through
masculine institutions: From discipline to protection to collaborative empowerment.
Criminology and Public Policy, *2*(2), 319–28.

Lynch, D. (2004). The protection, care and adjustment of refugee children in Australia,
15th International Conference on Child Abuse and Neglect. Brisbane.

Lynch, D. (2006). Cultural diversity in practice. In A. O'Hara and Z. Weber (eds), *Skills
for Human Service Practice: Working with Individuals, Groups and Communities*.
Melbourne: Oxford University Press.

Lynch, M. and Cunninghame, C. (2000). Understanding the needs of young asylum seekers. *Archives of Disease in Childhood*, *83*, 384–7.

Lynch, P. (2001). Keeping them home: The best interests of Indigenous children and communities in Canada and Australia. *Sydney Law Review*, *23*, 501–42.

Lyon, E. (2000). *Welfare, Poverty, and Abused Women: New Research and its
Implications*. Pennsylvania: National Resource Center on Domestic Violence.

Macaulay, T.B. (1906). *The History of England from thje Accession of James II*. London: Dent.

McClemens Report. (1961). *McClemens Royal Commission into Callan Park Mental
Hospital*. Canberra: Commonwealth Government of Australia.

McClennen, J. (2005). Domestic violence between same sex partners. *Journal of
Interpersonal Violence*, *20*(2), 149–54.

McCreadie, C. (1996). Elder abuse: An update on research [Electronic Version]. Retrieved
6 February 2007, from www.kcl.ac.uk/kis/schools/life_sciences/health/gerontology/pdf/
elderabus.html.

McDermott, J.M. and Garofalo, J. (2004). When advocacy for domestic violence victims
backfires. *Violence Against Women*, *10*(11), 1245–66.

Macdonald, G. (2001). *Effective Interventions for Child Abuse and Neglect: An Evidence-
Based Approach to Planning and Evaluating Interventions*. Chichester: John Wiley & Sons.

Macdonald, G. and Sirotich, F. (2005). Violence in the social work workplace: The
Canadian experience. *International Social Work*, *48*(6), 772–81.

McGregor, H. and Hopkins, A. (1991). *Working for Change: The Movement Against Domestic Violence.* Sydney: Allen and Unwin.

McInnes, E. (2004a). The impact of violence on mother's and children's needs during and after parental separation. *Early Child Development and Care, 174*(4), 367–8.

McInnes, E. (2004b, 1–3 November). *Keeping Children Safe: The Links Between Family Violence and Poverty. Conference paper presented to the Because Children Matter: Tackling Poverty Together.* Paper presented at the Uniting Missions National Conference, Adelaide.

McKelvey, R. and Webb, J. (1995). Unaccompained status as a risk factor in Vietnamese Americans. *Social Science Medicine, 41*(2), 261–6.

MacKinnon, C. (1982). Feminism, Marxism, Method and the State: An agenda for theory. *Signs: Journal of Women in Culture and Society, 7*(3), 532–58.

MacKinnon, L. (1992). *Child Abuse in Context: Participants views.* Unpublished PhD, University of Sydney, Sydney.

Macklin, M. (1997). Breaching the Idyll: Ideology, Intimacy and Social Service Provision in a Rural Community. In P. Share (ed.), *Communication and Culture in Rural Areas.* Wagga Wagga: Centre for Rural Social Research.

McLean, R. (2003). *Recovered, Not Cured.* Sydney: Allen and Unwin.

McNeill, P. (1998). *Counting the Rivers.* Adelaide: Wakefield Press.

Maddison, S. and Partridge, E. (2007). How Well Does Australian Democracy Serve Australian Women? In School of Social Sciences, Australian National University (ed.), *The Democratic Audit of Australia.* Canberra: The Australian National University.

Mahoney, M.R. (1991). Legal images of battered women: Redefining the issue of separation. *Michigan Law Review, 90*(1), 1–94.

Malcoe, L.H., Duran, B.M. and Montgomery, J.M. (2004). Socioeconomic disparities in intimate partner violence against Native American women: a cross-sectional study. *BMC Medicine, 2*(20).

Manne, R. and Corlett, D. (2004). Sending them home: Refugees and the new politics of indifference. *Quartley Essay* (13).

Manning, S. (1998). Empowerment in mental health programs: listening to the voices. In L.M. Gutierree, R.J. Parsons and E.O. Cox (eds), *Empowerment in Social Work Practice.* CA: Brooks/Cole.

Manning, S., Zibalese-Crawford, M. and Downey, E. (1994). *Colorado Mental Health Consumer and Family Development Project: Program Evaluation.* Denver, CO: University of Denver.

Mares, P. (2004). Asylum seekers: Australia's sledgehammer. *Australian Policy Online.*

Margolis, D. (1993). Women's movements around the world. *Gender and Society, 7*(3), 379–99.

Maris, R. (1991). Introduction to a special issue: Assessment and prediction of suicide. *Suicide and Life-Threatening Behaviour, 21,* 1–17.

Martin, G. (1998). Media influence to suicide: The search for solutions. *Archives of Suicide Research, 4,* 51–66.

Martin, J. (2006). Migrants and refugees. In W. Chui and J. Wilson (eds), *Social Work and Human Services Best Practice.* ? Melbourne: The Federation Press.

Mayhew, C. and Chappell, D. (2001). *Occupational Violence: Types, Reporting Patterns and Variations between Health Sectors. Papers Series No 139.* Sydney: Department of Industrial Relations UNSW Sydney.

Meadows, G., Singh, B. and Grigg, M. (2007). *Mental Health in Australia: Collaborative Community Practice* South Melboune: Oxford University Press.

Meares, R. (2006). Attacks on value: A new approach to depression. *Psychotherapy in Australia, 12*(3), 62–8.

Mears, J. (2003). Survival is not enough. *Violence Against Women. Violence Against Older Women in Australia, 19*(12), 1478–89.

Memmott, P. (1991). Queensland Aboriginal cultures and the deaths in custody victims. In L. Wyell (ed.), *Regional Report of Inquiry in Queensland: Royal Commission into Deaths in Custody* (pp. Appendix 2, 171–289). Canberra: Australian Government Publishing Service.

Memmott, P., Stacy, R., Chambers, C. and Keys, C. (2001). *Violence in Indigenous Communities: Report to the Crime Prevention Branch of the Attorney General's Department* Canberra: Commonwealth Attorney-General's Department.

Mendes, P. (2004). *Competing Visions of Community Development in Australia: Social Inclusion vs. Social Exclusion.* Paper presented at the Community Development Human Rights and the Grassroots Conference, Melbourne.

Mendes, P. and Moslehuddin, B. (2004). Graduating from the child welfare system: a comparison of the UK and Australian leaving care debates. *International Journal of Social Welfare, 13*, 322–39.

Merrill, G.S. (1996). Ruling the exceptions: Same sex battering and domestic violence theory. In C. Renzetti and C.H. Miley (eds), *Violence in Gay and Lesbian Partnerships* (pp. 9–23). New York Harrington Park Press.

Middleton, L. (1999). *Disabled Children: Challenging Social Exclusion.* Oxford: Blackwell Science.

Mikell, G. (1995). African Feminism: Toward a New Politics of Representation. *Feminist Studies, 21*, 405–24.

Millar, M. and Corby, B. (2006). The framework for the assessment of children in need and their families – A basis for 'therapeutic' encounter? *British Journal of Social Work, 36*, 887–99.

Miller, J. and Bell, C. (1996). Mapping men's mental health. *Journal of Community and Applied Social Psychology, 6*(5), 317–27.

Miller, S.L. (2001). The paradox of women arrested for domestic violence: Criminal justice professionals and service providers respond. *Violence Against Women, 7*(12), 1339–76.

Millett, K. (1970). *Sexual Politics.* New York: Double Day.

Millett, K. (1974). *Flying.* New York: Alfred A. Knopf.

Mills, L.G. (1999). Killing her softly: Intimate abuse and the violence of state intervention. *Harvard Law Review, 113*(2), 550–613.

Mills, L.G. (2003). *Insult to Injury: Rethinking our Responses to Intimate Abuse.* Princeton, NJ: Princeton University Press.

Mitchell, J. (1971). *Women's Estate.* New York: Pantheon Books.

Moe, A. and Bell, M. (2004). Abject economics: the effects of battering and violence on women's work and employability. *Violence Against Women, 10*(1), 29–55.

Mohanty, C. (1988). Under western eyes: Feminist scholarship and colonial discourses. *Feminist Review, 30*(Autumn), 61–83.

Mohanty, C. (2003). *Feminism Without Borders, Decolonizing Theory, Practicing Solidarity.* Durham and London: Duke University Press.

Mohanty, S., Sahu, G., Mohanty, M.K. and Patnaik, M. (2006). Suicide in India – A four year retrospective study. *Journal of Clinical Forensic Medicine,* doi:10.1016/j.jcfm. 2006.05.007.

Moracco, K.E., Runyan, C.W. and Loomis, D.P. (2000). Killed on the clock: a population-based study of workplace homicide, 1977–1991. *American Journal of Industrial Medicine, 37*(6), 629–36.

Moraga, C. and Anzaldua, G. (1983). *This Bridge Called My Back. Writings by Radical Women of Colour*. New York: Kitchen Table: Women of Color Press.

Moreton-Robinson, A. (2000). *Talkin' Up to the White Women: Indigenous Women and Feminism*. St Lucia: University of Queensland Press.

Morgan Disney and Associates. (2000). *Two Lives – Two Worlds. Older People and Domestic Violence*. Canberra: Parenerships Against Domestic Violence.

Morgan, R. (1978). *Going Too Far. The Personal Chronicle of a Feminist*. New York: Vintage Books.

Morrell, S., Page, A.N. and Taylor, R.J. (2006). The decline in Australian young male suicide. *Social Science & Medicine*, doi:10.1016/j.socscimed.2006.09.027.

Morris, J. (1996). *Encounters with Strangers: Feminism and Disability*. London: Women's Press.

Morrison, L. (2005). *Talking Back to Psychiatry: The Consumer/Survivor/Ex-patient Movement*. New York: Routledge.

Mukamal, K., Kawachi, I., Miller, M. and Rimm, E. (2007). Body mass index and risk of suicide among men [electronic version]. *Archives of Internal Medicine*, 167. Retrieved 14 March 2007, from http://www.archinternmed.com

Mullender, A. (1996). *Re-Thinking Domestic Violence: The Social Work and Probation Response*. London: Routledge.

Mullender, A. (2006). What children tell us. In C. Humphreys and J. Stanley (eds), *Domestic Violence and Child Protection: Directions for Good Practice* (pp. 53–68). London: Jessica Kingsley Publishers.

Mullender, A. and Hague, G. (2001). Women survivors' views. In J. Taylor-Browne (ed.), *What Works in Reducing Domestic Violence? A Comprehensive Guide for Professionals*. London: Whiting and Birch.

Mullender, A., Hague, G., Imam, U., Kelly, L., Malos, E. and Regan, L. (2002). *Children's Perspectives on Domestic Violence*. London: Sage.

Mullender, A. and Morley, R. (eds). (1994). *Children Living with Domestic Violence*. London: Birch and Whiting.

Munford, R. and Sanders, J. (1999). *Supporting Families*. Palmerston North, NZ: Dunmore Press.

Munro, E. (2005). A systems approach to investigating child abuse deaths. *British Journal of Social Work*, 35, 531–46.

Murphy, P.A. (1997). Recovering from the effects of domestic violence: Implications for welfare reform policy. *Law & Policy*, 19(2), 169–82.

Murray, S. (2005). An impossibly ambitious plan? Australian policy and the elimination of domestic violence. *Just Policy*, 38(December), 28–33.

Mythen, G. and Walklate, S. (2006). Introduction: Thinking beyond the risk society. In G. Mythen and S. Walklate (eds), *Beyond the Risk Society. Critical Reflecitons on Risk and Human Security* (pp. 1–7). Berkshire: Open University Press.

Nadien, M. (1996). Ageing women: Issues of mental health and maltreatment. In J.A. Sechzer, S.M. Pfafflin, E.L. Denmark, A. Griffin and S.S. Blumenthal (eds), *Women and Mental Health*. New York: New York Academy of Sciences.

Narayan, U. (1997). *Dislocating Cultures, Identities, Tradition and Third World Feminism*. London: Routledge.

National Occupational Health and Safety Commission (NOHSC). (1999). Program One Report: Occupational Violence. 51st meeting of NOHSC, 10 March 1999, Hobart.

National Practice Standard for the Mental Health Workforce. (2002). *Commonwealth Department of Health and Ageing*. Canberra: Publications Production Unit.

Naved, R.T. and Lars, P. (2005). Factors Associated with Spousal Physical Violence Against Women in Bangladesh. *Studies in Family Planning, 36*(4), 289–300.

Nelson, G. (1994). The development of a mental health coalition: A case study. *American Journal of Community Psychology, 22*(2), 229–55.

Nelson, G., Lord, J. and Ochocka, J. (2001). Empowerment and mental health in community: Narrative of psychiatric consumers/survivors. *Journal of Community Applied Social Psychology, 11*, 125–42.

Nelson, G., Ochocka, J., Griffin, K. and Lord, J. (1998). 'Nothing about me, without me': Participatory research with self-help/mutual aid organizations for psychiatric consumer/survivors. *American Journal of Community Psychology, 26*(6), 881–913.

NSW Bureau of Crime Statistics and Research. (2005). *NSW Recorded Crime Statistics 2005*. Sydney.

NSW Department of Community Services. (2006). *New South Wales Interagency Guidelines for Child Protection Intervention*. Sydney: NSW Department of Community Services.

NSW Department of Community Services. (2006). *Spotlight on Safety: Community attitudes to child protection, foster care and parenting*. Sydney: NSW Department of Community Services.

NSW Department of Ageing, Disability and Home Care Services. (2007). *Draft New South Wales Interagency Protocol for Responding to Abuse of Older People*. Sydney: NSW Government.

NSW Department of Health. (2004). Suicide Risk Assessment and Management Protocols: Community Mental Health Service. Sydney: NSW Department of Health.

NSW Department of Health. (2006). *A Statewide Approach to Measuring and Responding to Consumer Perceptions and Experiences of Adult Mental Health Services: A Report on Stage One of the Development of the MH-CoPES Framework and Questionnaires*. Sydney: NSW Department of Health.

NSW Domestic Violence Committee. (1989). *NSW Domestic Violence Committee Report 1985–1988*. Sydney: Women's Co-ordination Unit.

NSW Government. (2006). *New South Wales Interagency Guidelines for Child Protection Intervention*. Sydney: NSW Government.

NSW Government's Child Protection Senior Officers Group (CPSOG). (2006). New South Wales Interagency Guidelines for Child Protection Intervention: NSW Government.

NSW Health. (2005). Zero Tolerance Response to Violence in the New South Wales Health Workplace. Policy Directive PD2005_315: New South Wales Government.

NSW Health Department. (1992). *NSW Aboriginal Family Health Strategy*. North Sydney: NSW Health Department.

NSW Health Department. (2002). *Aboriginal Family Health Strategy*. North Sydney: NSW Health Department.

NSW Law Reform Commission. (1997). *The Aboriginal Child Placement Principle, Research Report No. 7*. Sydney: NSW Law Reform Commission.

NSW Ombudsman. (2006). *Domestic violence: improving police practice*. Sydney.

NSW Ombudsman. (2006). *NSW Ombudsman Report of Reviewable deaths in 2005. Volume 2: Child Deaths*. Sydney.

O'Hagan, K. and Dillenburger, K. (1995). *The Abuse of Women within Childcare Work*. Buckingham: Open University Press.

Ocana-Riola, R. and Sanchez-Cantalejo, C. (2005). Rurality index for small areas in Spain. *Social Indicators Research, 73*, 247–66.

O'Connor, K. and Rowe, J. (2005). Elder abuse. *Reviews in Clinical Gerontology, 15*, 47–54.

Office of Women's Policy. (2005). Safe at work? Women's experience of violence in the workplace. Summary report of research undertaken by Office of Women's Policy Melbourne. Melbourne: Department for Victorian Communities.

Oliver, I. (2001). 'Two hats: A cautionary tale'. In G. Meadows and B. Singh (eds), *Mental Health in Australia*. South Melbourne: Oxford University Press.

Oliver, M. (1996). *Understanding Disability: From Theory to Practice*. Basingstoke: Macmillan.

Oliver, M. and Sapey, B. (2006). *Social Work with Disabled People* (3rd edn). Basingstoke: Palgrave Macmillan.

Olmstead. (1999). Supreme Court Upholds ADA 'Integration Mandate' in Olmstead decision. Retrieved 8 December 2006, from http:www.accessiblesociety.org/topics/ada/olmsteadoverview.htm

Olsen, A. and Epstein, M. (2001). The consumer of mental health services: Consumers and services. In G. Meadows and B. Singh (eds), *Mental Health in Australia* (pp. 138–41). South Melbourne: Oxford University Press.

Onyx, J., and Bullen, P. (2000). Measuring social capital in five communities. *Journal of Applied Behavioural Sciences, 36*(1), 23–42.

O'Shane, P. (1976). Is there any relevance in the women's movement for Aboriginal women? *Refractory Girl, September*, 31–5.

Owens, D., Horrocks, J. and House, A. (2002). Fatal and non-fatal repetition of self-harm. *British Journal of Psychiatry, 181*, 193–9.

Padgett, D.K., Burns, B.J., and Grau, L.A. (1998). Risk factors and resilience: Mental health needs and service use of older women. In B.L. Levin, A.K. Blanch and A. Jennings (eds), *Women's Mental Health Services: Public Health Perspective* (pp. 390–413). Thousand Oaks: Sage.

Page, J. (2006, 9 October). Elderly suffer abuse as old ways change. *The Times*.

Papillion, M. (2002). Immigration, diversity and social inclusion in Canada's cities. *Canadian Policy Research Networks Inc*. Retrieved 15 December 2004, from http://www.cprn.org

Pardeck, J. (1989). *Child Abuse and Neglect: Theory, Research and Practice* New York: Gordon & Breach Scoence Publishers.

Partnerships Against Domestic Violence. (2003). Domestic violence: Working with men, phase One meta evaluation report. Canberra: Office of Status of Women, Department of Prime Minister and Cabinet, Commonwealth Government.

Peace, S., Kellaher, L. and Willcocks, D. (1997). *Re-evaluating Residential Care*. Buckingham: Open University Press.

Pearson, N. (2000). *Dysfunctional Society and Aboriginal Issues*. Ben Chifley Memorial Lecture, Bathurst.

Pease, B. (2003). Men and masculinities: Profeminist approaches to changing men. In J. Allan, B. Pease and L. Briskman (eds), *Critical Social Work*. London: Allen and Unwin.

Pease, B. and Camilleri, P. (eds). (2001) *Working with Men in the Human Services*. Sydney: Allen and Unwin.

Pecora, P.J., McAuley, C. and Rose, W. (2006). Effectiveness of child welfare interventions. In C. McAuley, P.J. Pecora and W. Rose (eds), *Enhancing the Well-being of Children and Families through Effective Interventions. International Evidence for Practice* (pp. 14–20). London: Jessica Kingsley Publishers.

Pecora, P.J., Whittaker, J.K. and Maluccio, A.N. (2006). Child welfare in the US. In C. McAuley, P.J. Pecora and W. Rose (eds), *Enhancing the Well-being of Children and Families through Effective Interventions*. London: Jessica Kingsley Publishers.

Pedersen, D. (2002). Political violence, ethnic conflict and contemporary wars: Broad implications for health and social well-being. *Social Science and Medicine, 55*, 175–90.

Peel, M. (2003). *The Lowest Rung: Voices of Australian Poverty*. Melbourne: Cambridge University Press.

Peetz, D. (2006). *Brave New Workplace: How Individual Contracts are Changing our Jobs*. Sydney: Allen and Unwin.

Peetz, D. (2007). *Brave New Work Choices: What is the Story So Far?* Paper presented at the 24th conference of the Association of Industrial Relations Academics of Australia and New Zealand, Auckland, NZ.

Peirce, J. (2005). *Family Violence and the Law: Putting 'Private' Violence on the Public Agenda*. Paper presented at the Families Matter: 9th Australian Institute of Family Studies Conference, Melbourne, Victoria.

Pence, E.L. and McDonnell, C. (1999). Developing policies and protocols. In M.F. Shepard and E.L. Pence (eds), *Coordinating Community Responses to Domestic Violence: Lessons from Duluth and Beyond* (pp. 41–64). Thousand Oaks, CA: Sage.

Penhale, B. (2003). Older women, domestic violence and elder abuse: A review of commonalities, differences and shared approaches. *Journal of Elder Abuse & Neglect, 15*(3/4), 163–83.

Perlesz, A. (1999). Complex responses to trauma: Challenges in bearing witness. *The Australian and New Zealand Journal of Family Therapy, 20*(1), 11–19.

Peter, T. (2006). Domestic violence in the United States and Sweden: A welfare state typology comparison within a power resources framework. *Womens Studies International Forum, 29*(1), 96–107.

Pewewardy, N. (2004). The political is personal: The essential obligation of white feminist family therapists to deconstruct white privilege. *Journal of Feminist Family Therapy, 16*(1), 53–67.

Phillips, R. (2004). From waves of action to the 'dead calm' responses to violence against women in the new millennium. *Women in Welfare Education, 7*, 17–32.

Phillips, R. (2006a). Undoing an activist response: feminism and the Australian government's domestic violence policy. *Critical Social Policy, 26*(1), 192–219.

Phillips, R. (2006b). Women and poverty: The application of feminism in overcoming women's poverty in the global context. In K. Serr (ed.), *Thinking About Poverty* (3rd edn (pp. 25–34). Sydney: The Federation Press.

Phillips, R. and Kendig, H. (forthcoming, June 2007). Health, economic, and policy implications of an ageing Australia. In R. Phillips (ed.), *Generational Change and New Policy Challenges: Australia and South Korea* (pp. 701–20). Sydney: University of Sydney Press.

Pilgrim, D. and Hitchman, L. (1999). User involvement in mental health service development. In C. Newnes, G. Holmes and C. Dunn (eds), *This is Madness: A Critical Look at Psychiatry and the Future of the Mental Health Services*. Ross-on-Wye: PCCS Books.

Pilgrim, D. and Rogers, A. (1999). *A Sociology of Mental Health and Illness* (2nd ed.). Buckingham: Open University Press.

Pinheiro, P.S. (2006). *Violence Against Children*: United Nations.

Pockett, R. (2003). Staying in hospital social work. *Social Work in Health Care, 36*(3), 1–23.

Poiner, G. (1990). *The Good Old Rule. Gender and Other Power Relationships in a Rural Community*. Sydney: Sydney University Press.

Poustie, A. and Neville, R. (2004). Deliberate self-harm cases: a primary care perspective. *Nursing Standard*, *18*(48), 33–6.

Powers, L., Ward, N., Ferris, L., Nelis, T., Ward, M., Wieck, C., et al. (2002). Leadership by people with disabilities in self-determination systems changing. *Journal of Disability Policy Studies*, *13*(2), 125–9.

Poynter, B., and Warne, C. (1988). *Preventing Violence to Staff*. London: HSE Books.

Puckett, T. and Cleak, H. (1994). Caution – helping may be hazardous: Client abuse, threats and assaults. *Australian Social Work*, *47*(1), 3–9.

Pugh, R. (2003). Considering the countryside: Is there a case for rural social work? *British Journal of Social Work*, *33*, 67–85.

Putt, J. and Higgins, K. (1997). *Violence Against Women in Australia: Key Research and Data Issues*. Canberra: Australian Institute of Criminology.

Queensland Domestic Violence Task Force. (1988). *Beyond These Walls: Report of the Queensland Domestic Violence Task Force to the Minister for Family Services and Welfare Housing*. Brisbane: Queensland. Department of Family Services.

Radford, L. and Hester, M. (2006). *Mothering Through Domestic Violence*. London: Jessica Kingsley Publishers.

Rains, S. (2001). *Don't Suffer in Silence: Building an Effective Response to Bullying at Work*. In N. Tehrani (ed.), *Building a Culture of Respect*. London: Taylor and Francis.

Raphael, J. (2004). Rethinking criminal justice responses to intimate partner violence. *Violence Against Women*, *10*(11), 1354–66.

Rappaport, J. (1993). Narrative studies: Personal stories and identity transformation in the mutual help context. *Journal of Applied Behavioral Science*, *29*, 239–56.

Rappaport, J. (1995). Empowerment meets narrative: Listening to stories and creating settings. *American Journal of Community Psychology*, *23*, 795–807.

Raue, P. and Brown, E. (2006). Strategies for assessing suicidal ideation. *Psychotherapy in Australia*, *13*(1), 70–4.

Rawsthorne, M. (2003). Social work and the prevention of sexual violence in rural communities. The ties that bind. *Rural Social Work*, *8*(3), 4–11.

Rawsthorne, M. (2006). Instability among low income families. *Just Policy*, *40*, 25–31.

Read, J. and Reynolds, J. (1996). *Speaking Our Minds: An Anthology of Personal Experiences of Mental Distress and Its Consequences*. London: Macmillan.

Refugee Council of Australia. (2007). Australia's refugee programs. Retrieved 3 February 2007, from HTTP: www.refugeecouncil.org.au/arp/stats-02.html.

Reid, C. and Tom, A. (2006). Poor women's discourses of legitimacy, poverty and health. *Gender and Society*, *20*(3), 402–21.

Renzetti, C.M. (1992). *Violent Betrayal: Partner Abuse in Lesbian Relationships*. Newbury Park: Sage.

Renzetti, C.M. (1999). The challenges posed by women's use of violence in intimate relationships. In S. Lamb (ed.), *New Versions of Victims: Feminists Struggle with the Concept* (pp. 42–56). New York: New York University Press.

Republic of Uganda Ministry of Finance Planning and Economic Development. (2006). *Uganda National Report for the Implementation of the Programme of Action for the Least Developed Countries for the Decade 2001–2010. Submitted to the United Nations Office of the High Representative for the Least Developed Countries and Small Island Developing States (UN-OHRLLS)*.

Reynolds, H. (2000). *Why Weren't We told? A Personal Search for the Truth About Our History*. Australia: Penguin Books.

Rich, A. (1980). Compulsory heterosexuality. *Signs: Journal of Women in Culture and Society*, *5*, 631–60.

Richardson, S. and Asthana, S. (2006). Inter-agency information sharing in health and social care services: The role of professional culture. *British Journal of Social Work*, *36*, 657–69.

Riley, A. (1996). Murder and social work. *Australian Social Work*, *49*(2), 37–43.

Ristock, J.L. (2002). *No More Secrets: Violence in Lesbian Relationships*. New York, London: Routledge.

Robb, B. (1967). *Sans Everything: A Case to Answer*. London: Nelson.

Roberson, M. (2007 personal communication). Revised Interagency Protocol for Responding to Abuse of Older People (NSW Department of Ageing Disability and Home Care).

Roberts, G.L. (2000). Evaluating the prevalence and impact of domestic violence. In A. Shalev, R.R. Yehuda and A. McFarlane (eds), *International Handbook of Human Responses to Trauma*. New York: Kluwer Academic/Plenum Publishers.

Robinson, A.L. and Stroshine, M.S. (2005). The importance of expectation fulfilment on domestic violence victims' satisfaction with the police in the UK. *Policing: An International Journal of Police Strategies & Management*, *28*(2), 301–20.

Rogers, A. and Pilgrim, D. (1993). Service users' views of psychiatric treatments. *Sociology of Health and Illness*, *15*, 612–31.

Rogers, A. and Pilgrim, D. (2001). *Mental Health Policy in Britain: A Critical Introduction*. Basingstoke: Palgrave Macmillan.

Romkens, R. (2006). Protecting prosecution: Exploring the powers of law in an intervention program for domestic violence. *Violence Against Women*, *12*(2), 160–86.

Rose, S.M. and Black, B. (1985). *Advocacy and Empowerment: Mental Health Care in the Community*. New York: Routledge and Kegan Paul.

Rose, S.M. and Black, B. (1990). Advocacy/empowerment: An approach to clinical practice for social work. *Journal of Sociology and Social Welfare*, *17*(2), 41–52.

Rose, W., Gray, J. and McAuley, C. (2006). Child welfare in the UK: Legislation, policy and practice. In C. McAuley, P.J. Pecora and W. Rose (eds), *Enhancing the Well-being of Children and Families through Effective Interventions* (pp. 21–32). London: Jessica Kingsley Publishers.

Rousseau, C. and Drapeau, A. (2003). Are refugee children an at-risk group? *Journal of Refugee Studies*, *16*(1), 67–81.

Rousseau, C., Drapeau, A., Lacroix, L., Bagilishya, D. and Heusch, N. (2005). Evaluation of a classroom program of creative expression workshops for refugee and immigrant children. *Journal of Child Psychology and Psychiatry*, *46*(2), 180–5.

Rowbottom, S. (1973). *Women's Consciousness Men's World*. Baltimore: Penguin.

Royal Australian and New Zealand College of Psychiatrists. (2005). Self-harm: Australian treatment guide for consumers and carers [Electronic Version]. Retrieved 18 December 2006, from https://www.ranzcp.org/pdffiles/cpgs/AUS_CPGs/Self%20harm%20(Aus).pdf.

Russell, D. (1995). *Women, Madness and Medicine*. Cambridge: Polity Press.

Rutter, M. (1987). Psychological resilience and protective mechanisms. *American Journal of Orthopsychiatry*, *57*, 316–31.

Saleebey, D. (1992). Introduction: Power in the people. In D. Saleebey (ed.), *The Strengths Perspective in Social Work Practice*. New York: Longman.

Saleebey, D. (1996). The strengths perspective in social work practice. Extensions and cautions. *Social Work*, *41*(3), 296–305.

Sales, R. (2002). The deserving and the undeserving? Refugees, asylum seekers and welfare in Britain. *Critical Social Policy*, *22*(3), 456–78.

Sartorius, N. (1999). One of the last obstacles to better mental health care: The stigma of mental illness. In J. Guimon, W. Fischer and N. Sartorius (eds), *The Image of Madness*. Basel: Karger.

Sartorius, N. and Schulz, H. (2005). *Reducing the Stigma of Mental Illness: A Report from the Global Programme of the World Psychiatric Association*. Cambridge: Cambridge University Press.

Sawer, M. (2003). The Life and Times of Women's Policy Machinery in Australia. In S. Rai (ed.), *Mainstreaming Gender, Democratizing the State? International Mechanisms for the Advancement of Women*. Manchester: Manchester University Press.

Sayers, J. (1986). Violence and social work. *Australian Social Work*, *39*(1), 5–11.

Scalora, M.J., Washington, D.O. and Casady, T. (2003). Nonfatal workplace violence risk factors: data from a police contact sample. *Journal of Interpersonal Violence*, *18*(3), 310–27.

Schaeffer, J. (1999). Older and isolated women and domestic violence project. *Journal of Elder Abuse & Neglect*, *11*(1), 59–77.

Schechter, S. (2000). *Expanding Solutions for Domestic Violence and Poverty: What Battered Women with Abused Children Need from their Advocates*. Pennsylvania: National Resource Center on Domestic Violence.

Schneider, E.M. (1992). Particularity and generality: Challenges of feminist theory and practice in work on woman-abuse. *New York University Law Review*, *67*, 520–68.

Schroder-Butterfill, E. and Marianti, R. (2006). A framework for understanding old-age vulnerabilities. *Ageing & Society*, *26*, 9–35.

Schulman, M.D. and Anderson, C. (1999). The dark side of the force: A case study of restructuring and social captial. *Rural Sociology*, *64*(3), 351–72.

Scott, D. (2006). Towards a public health model of child protection in Australia. *Communities, Families and Children Australia*, *1*(1), 10–16.

Scott, E.K., London, A.S. and Myers, N.A. (2002). Dangerous dependencies: The intersection of welfare reform and domestic violence. *Gender & Society*, *16*(6), 878–97.

Scourfield, J. (2003). *Gender and Child Protection*. Basingstoke: Palgrave/Macmillan.

Scutt, J. (2006). Medico-legal issues: when women speak into silence. In G. Roberts, K. Hegarty and G. Feder (eds), *Intimate Partner Abuse Health Professionals: New Approaches to Domestic Violence* (pp. 163–77). Edinburgh: Churchill Livingstone Elsevier.

Seabrook, J. (2000). *No Hiding Place: Child Sex Tourism and the Role of Extraterritorial Legislation*. London: Zed Books.

Segal, S., Silverman, C. and Temkin, T. (1993). Empowerment and self-help agency practice for people with mental disabilities. *Social Work*, *38*(6), 705–12.

Sen, A. (1999). *Development as Freedom*. New York: Oxford University Press.

Sen, A. (2006). *Identity and Violence: The Illusion of Destiny*. New York: W.W. Norton.

Senate Community Affairs Reference Committee (SCARC). (2004). *A Hand Up Not a Hand Out: Report on Poverty and Financial Hardship*. Canberra: Commonwealth of Australia.

September, R. (2006). The progress of child protection in South Africa. *International Journal of Social Welfare*, *15*(S1), S65–S72.

Share, P. (1997). Beyond 'Country Mindedness': Representations in the Post-rural Era. In P. Share (ed.), *Communication and Culture in Rural Areas*. Wagga Wagga: Centre for Rural Social Research.

Shneidman, E. (1987). Approaches and commonalities of suicide. In R. Diekstra (ed.), *Attitudinal Factors in Suicidal Behavior and its Prevention*. Leiden: Swets & Zeitlinger/Brill.

Shneidman, E. and Mandelkorn, P. (1994). Some facts and fables of suicide. In E. Shneidman, N. Farberow and R. Litman (eds), *The Psychology of Suicide: A Clinician's Guide to Evaluation and Treatment*. New Jersey: Jason Aronson.

Shortall, S. (2004). Social and economic goals – civic inclusion or exclusion? An analysis of rural development theory and practice. *Journal of the European Society for Rural Sociology*, *44*(1), 109–23.

Silove, D., Steel, Z. and Watters, C. (2000). Policies of deterrence and the mental health of asylum seekers. *Journal of the American Medical Association*, *284*, 604–11.

Simpson, E.L. and House, A.O. (2002). Involving users in the delivery and evaluation of mental health services: Systemic review. *British Medical Journal*, *325*, 1265–7.

Simpson, J., Hornby, G., Davis, L. and Murray, R. (2005). Positive parent–professional relationship: Allies who emancipate one another. In P. O'Brien and M. Sullivan (eds), *Allies in Emancipation: Shifting from Providing Service to Being of Support*. South Melbourne: Thomson.

Smart, C. (1989). *Feminism and the Power of the Law*. London: Routledge.

Smith, M. (2006). Early interventions with young children and their parents in the UK. In C. McAuley, P.J. Pecora and W. Rose (eds), *Enhancing the Well-being of Children and Families through Effective Interventions* (pp. 46–57). London: Jessica Kingsley Publishers.

Smokowski, P. (1998). Prevention and intervention strategies for promoting resilience in disadvantaged children. *Social Science Review*, *72*(3), 337–64.

Snider, L. (1998). Towards safer societies: Punishment, masculinities and violence against women. *The British Journal of Criminology*, *38*(1), 1–39.

Somer, E., Buchbinder, E., Peled-Avram, M. and Ben -Yzhack, Y. (2004). The stress and coping of Israeli emergency room social workers following terrorist attacks. *Qualitative Health Research*, *14*(8), 1077–93.

South East Wales Executive Group for the Protection of Vulnerable Adults. (2003). *Protecting Vulnerable Adults*. Cardiff: South East Wales Executive Group for the Protection of Vulnerable Adults.

Spratt, T. (2001). The influence of child protection orientation on child welfare practice. *British Journal of Social Work*, *31*, 933–54.

Spring, N. and Stern, M. (1998). Nurses and workplace violence: Nurse abuse? Couldn't Be!' *Nurse Advocate*, Ohio Health Care Network.

Spring, N. and Stern, M. (1999). Intraprofessional abuse and violence in the nursing workplace. *Nurse Advocate*, Ohio Health Care Network.

Stacey, J. (1986). Are feminists afraid to leave the home? In J. Mitchell and A. Oakley (eds), *What Is Feminism?* (pp. 219–48). Oxford: Basil Blackwell.

Stamatopoulu, E. (1995). Women's rights and the United Nations. In J. Peters and A. Wolper (eds), *Women's Rights Human Rights, International Feminist Perspectives* (pp. 36–48). New York: Routledge.

Standing Committee on Aboriginal and Torres Strait Islander Health and Statistical Information Management Committee. (2006). National summary of the 2003 and 2004 jurisdictional reports against the Aboriginal and Torres Strait Islander health performance indicators: AIHW cat. no. IHW 16. Retrieved 24 April 2007, from http://www.aihw.gov.au/publications/ihw/ns03-04jratsihpi/ ns03-04jratsihpi.pdf

Stanley, J. and Goddard, C. (2002). *In the Firing Line. Violence and Power in Child Protection Work*. Chichester: John Wiley and Sons.

Stanley, N., Penhale, B., Riordan, D., Barbour, R. and Holden, S. (2003). *Child Protection and Mental Health Services. Interprofessional Responses to the Needs of Mothers*. Bristol: The Policy Press.

Stark, E. (2004). Insults, injury, and injustice. *Violence Against Women, 10*(11), 1302–30.

Stewart, S. (2005). Suicidality, interpersonal trauma and cultural diversity: a review of the literature. *Australian e-Journal for the Advancement of Mental Health, 4*(2).

Stewart, S. (2006). *Suicidality, Interpersonal Trauma and Cultural Diversity Project: Final Report*. Parramatta BC: Education Centre Against Violence.

Stewart, S., Manion, I. and Davidson, S. (2002). Emergency management of the adolescent suicide attempter: A review of the literature. *Journal of Adolescent Health, 30*, 312–25.

Stilwell, F. (2006). Processes of globalisation: The generation of wealth and poverty. In K. Serr (ed.), *Thinking About Poverty* (3rd edn). Sydney: The Federation Press.

Suicide Prevention Australia. (2006). A blue print for the future: Developing a national vision. Sydney: Suicide Prevention Australia.

Sullivan, C.M. and Bybee, D.I. (1999). Reducing violence using community-based advocacy for women with abusive partners. *Journal of Consulting and Clinical Psychology, 67*(1), 43–53.

Sullivan, M. and Munford, R. (2005). Disability and support: The interface between disability theory and support – and individual challenge. In P. O'Brien and M. Sullivan (eds), *Allies in Emancipation: Shifting from Providing Service to Being of Support*. South Melbourne: Thomson.

Sultan, A. and O'Sullivan, K. (2001). Psychological disturbances in asylum seekers held in long term detention: a participant-observer account. *Medical Journal of Australia 175*, 593–6.

Summers, A. (1975). *Damned Whores and God's Police. The Colonisation of Women in Australia*. London: Allen Lane.

Support Coalition International. (2000). The Highlander call for action. *Dendron, 43*(5).

Sutherland, S. (1976). *Breakdown*. London: Weidenfeld and Nicolson.

Swan, P. and Raphael, B. (1995). *Ways Forward: National Consultancy Project on Aboriginal and Torres Strait Islander Mental Health*. Canberra: Australian Government Publishing Service.

Swanberg, J., Logan, T. and Macke, M. (2005). Intimate partner violence, employment, and the workplace: Consequences and future directions. *Trauma, Violence & Abuse, 6*(4), 286–312.

Szasz, T. (1961). *The Myth of Mental Illness*. New York: Harper and Row.

Taft, A. (2003). *Promoting Women's Mental Health: The Challenge of Intimate/Domestic Violence Against Women*: Australian Domestic and Family Violence Clearinghouse.

Tascon, S. (2002). Refugees and asylum seekers in Australia: border crossers of the postcolonial imaginary [Electronic Version]. *Australian Journal of Human Rights*. Retrieved 7 February 2007, from http://bar.austlii.edu.au/au/journals/AJHR/2002/9.html

Tatz, C. (1991). Australia's genocide: 'They soon forget their offspring'. *Social Education, 55*(2), 97–8.

Taylor, B. (2006). Risk management paradigms in health and social services for professional decision making on the long-term care of older people. *British Journal of Social Work, 36*, 1411–29.

Taylor, J., Cheers, B., Wetra and Gentle, I. (2004). Supporting community solutions to family violence. *Australian Social Work, 57*(1) 71–83.

Taylor, J. and Stanovic, D. (2005). *Refugees and Regional Settlement: Balancing Priorities*. Melbourne: Brotherhood of St Lawrence.

Tehrani, N. (2004). *Workplace Trauma: Concepts, Assessment and Interventions*. New York: Brunner-Routledge.

Terzieff, J. (2002). Pakistan's fiery shame: Women die in stove deaths. *Women's E-News*. Retrieved 5 February 2007, from http://www.womensenews.org/article.cfm/dyn/aid/1085/context/cover/

Tester, F.J. and McNicoll, P. (2004). Isumagijaksaq: mindful of the state: social constructions of Inuit suicide. *Social Science & Medicine, 58*(12), 2625–36.

The Editor's Choice. (30 November, 2002). *British Medical Journal, 325*.

Thomas, P. (1996). Big boys don't cry? Mental health and the politics of gender. *Journal of Mental Health, 5*(2), 107–10.

Thomas, S., Thomas, S., Nafees, B. and Bhugra, D. (2004). I was running away from death' – the pre-flight experiences of unaccompanied asylum seeking children in the UK. *Child Care, Health and Development, 30*(2), 113–22.

Thompson, D. (2001). *Radical Feminism Today*. London: Sage.

Thompson, N. (2006). *Anti-Discriminatory Practice* (4th edn). Basingstoke: Palgrave Macmillan.

Tolman, R.M. and Raphael, J. (2000). A review of research on welfare and domestic violence. *Journal of Social Issues, 56*(4), 655–82.

Tomison, A. (2002, 2–4 September). *Evidence-based practice in child protection: What do we know and how do we better inform practice*. Paper presented at the What Works? Evidence Based Practice in Child and family Services, Bondi Beach, NSW.

Tomita, S. (2006). Mistreated and negelected elders. In B. Berkman and S. D'Ambruoso (eds), *Handbook of Social Work in Health and Aging*. Oxford: Oxford University Press.

Tönnies, F. (1957). *Gemeinschaft und Gessellschaft*. Trans and ed. C.P. Loomis. East Lansing: Michigan State University Press.

Tousignant, M., Mishara, B.L., Caillaud, A., Fortin, V. and St-Laurent, D. (2005). The impact of media coverage of the suicide of a well-known Quebec reporter: the case of Gaetan Girouard. *Social Science & Medicine, 60*(9), 1919–26.

Tregeagle, S. (1990). *Poverty and the Abuse and Neglect of Children, Monograph 12*. Sydney: Barnardos Australia.

Trickett, E. (2006). *They Couldn't Hear Me Scream: Women 45 Years and Over and Homelessness in Rural South Australia*. University of South Australia, Adelaide.

Trimboli, L. and Bonney, R. (1997). An Evaluation of the NSW Apprehended Violence Order Scheme. Retrieved 19 September 2006, from http://www.lawlink.nsw.gov.au/lawlink/bocsar/ll_ bocsar.nsf/vwFiles/L11.pdf/$file/L11.pdf.

Tsun On-Kee, A. (2006, 13 October). *The Landscape of Domestic Violence: Our Choice is to Frame and Picture it*. Paper presented at the Symposium on Domestic Violence – Welfare of Children and Families, Baptist University Hong Kong.

Tucci, J., Mitchell, J. and Goddard, C. (2006). *Every Child Needs a Hero: A Report Tracking Australian Children's Concerns and Attitudes About Childhood*. Melbourne: Australian Childhood Foundation.

United Nations: Universal Declaration of Human Rights, Article 14. Retrieved on 27 July 2007, from: http://idir.net/~cnc/UN_UDRH.htm

UNICEF. (2006). *The State of the World's Children 2007: Women and Children. The Double Dividend of Gender Equality*.

United Nations Children's Fund (UNICEF). (2007a). *Child Poverty in Perspective: An Overview of Child Well-being in Rich Countries*. Florence: UNICEF Innocenti Research Centre.

United Nations Children's Fund (UNICEF). (2007b). *The State of the World's Children 2007. Women and Children: The Double Dividend of Gender Equality*. Florence: UNICEF Innocenti Research Centre.

United Nations Development Programme (UNDP). (2005). *Human Development Report 2005*. New York: Oxford University Press.

Ursel, J. (2002). 'His sentence is my freedom': Processing domestic violence cases in the Winnipeg Family Violence Court. In L. Tutty and C. Goard (eds), *Reclaiming Self: Issues and Resources for Women Abused by Intimate Partners* (pp. 43–63): Fernwood Publishing.

Ussher, J.M. (1991). *Women's Madness: Misogyny or Mental Illness?* Amherst: University of Massachusetts Press.

van Eyk, H., and Baum, F. (2002). Learning about interagency collaboration: Trialling collaborative projects between hospitals and community health services. *Health and Social care in the Community*, *10*(4), 262–9.

Van Hightower, N. and Gorton, J. (2002). A Case Study of Community-based Responses to Rural Woman Battering. *Violence Against Women*, *8*(7), 845–72.

Van Hightower, N.R., Gorton, J. and DeMoss, C.L. (2000). Predictive models of domestic violence and fear of intimate partners among migrant and seasonal farm worker women. *Journal of Family Violence*, *15*(2), 137–54.

Vasta, E. (2004). Community, the state and the deserving citizen: Pacific Islanders in Australia. *Journal of Ethnic and Migration Studies*, *30*(1), 195–214.

Vetten, L. (2005). 'Show Me the Money': A Review of Budgets Allocated Towards Implementation of South Africa's Domestic Violence Act. *Politikon*, *32*, 277–95.

Victorian Health Promotion Foundation. (2004). *The Health Costs of Violence: Measuring the Burden of Disease Caused by Intimate Partner Violence. A Summary of Findings*. Melbourne: Mental Health Promotion Foundation.

Vinson, T. (2007). *Dropping off the Edge: The Distribution of Disadvantage in Australia*. Victoria: Jesuit Social Services/Catholic Social Services Australia.

Vinton, L. (2003). A model collaborative project toward making domestic violence centres elder ready. *Violence Against Women*, *19*(12), 1504–13.

Wacogne, I. (2003). Desperately 'seeking asylum', Postcard from Down Under [Electronic Version]. *Archives of Disease in Childhood*, 239. Retrieved December 11 2006 from http://www.unesco. org/most/apmrnwp5.htm

Walby, C. (1990). *Theorising Patriarchy*. Oxford: Blackwell.

Walby, S. and Allen, J. (2004). *Domestic Violence, Sexual Assault and Stalking: Findings from the British Crime Survey*. London: Home Office.

Waldfogel, J. (1998). Re-thinking the paradigm for child protection. *The Future of Children: Protecting Children from Abuse and Neglect*, *8*(1), 104–19.

Walker, G. (1990). *Family Violence and the Women's Movement*. Toronto: University of Toronto Press.

Walker, L.E. (1984). The *Battered Woman Syndrome*. New York: Springer Publishing Co.

Walker, L.E. (1977–8). Battered Women and Learned Helplessness. *Victimology*, *2*(3–4), 525–34.

Walker, S. and Matin, I. (2006). Changes in the lives of the ultra poor: an exploratory study. *Development in Practice*, *16*(1), 80–4.

Wallcraft, J. and Michaelson, J. (2002). Developing a survivor discourse to replace the 'psychopathology' of breakdown and crisis. In C. Newnes, G. Holmes and C. Dunn (eds), *This is Madness*. Llangarron: PCCS Books.

Wallis J. and Dollery, B. (2002). Social capital and local government capacity. *Australian Journal of Public Administration, 61*(3), 76–85.

Wang Lih-Rong. (2006, 13 October). *Help-Seeking Behaviour of Intimate Partner's Violence: The Reality and Its Implications.* Paper presented at the Symposium on Domestic Violence – Welfare of Children and Families, Baptist University Hong Kong.

Wappett, T. (2002). Self-determination and disability rights: Lessons from the women's movement. *Journal of Disability Policy Studies, 13*(2), 119–24.

Ward, C. (1997). Culture learning, acculturative stress, and psychopathology; three perspectives on acculturation. *Applied Psychology: An International Review, 46*(1), 58–62.

Waterson, J. (1999). Redefining community care social work: needs or risks led? *Health and Social care in the Community, 7*(4), 276–9.

Watson, G. (2001). A critical response to the Keys Young Report: Ending domestic violence? Programs for perpetrators. *Australian and New Zealand Journal of Family Therapy, 22*(2), 91–5.

Watson, G. and Williams, J. (1992). Feminist practice in therapy. In J. Ussher and P. Nicolson (eds), *Gender Issues in Clinical Psycholgy.* London: Routledge.

Watts, C. and Zimmerman, C. (2002). Violence against women: global scope and magnitude. *The Lancet, 359*(9313), 1232–7.

Waugh, F. (1997). *Policy in Action: An Exploration of Practice by Front-Line Workers in the New South Wales Department of Community Services, in Responding to Notifications of Child Emotional Abuse.* Unpublished PhD, University of Sydney, Sydney.

Waugh, F. (2006). Risk assessment: Working within a legal framework. In A. O'Hara and Z. Weber (eds), *Skills for Human Service Practice: Working with Individuals, Groups and Communities* (pp. 86–98). Melbourne: Oxford University Press.

Way, I., VanDeusen, K., Martin, G., Applegate, B. and Jandle, D. (2004). Vicarious trauma: a comparison of clinicians who treat survivors of sexual abuse and sexual offenders. *Journal of Interpersonal Violence, 19*(1), 49–71.

Weber, Z. (2005). Case management research. Unpublished.

Weber, Z. and Bugarszki, Z. (2007). Some reflections on social workers' perspectives on mental health services in two Cities: Sydney, Australia and Budapest, Hungary. *International Social Work, 50*(2), 145–55.

Websdale, N. (1995). Rural woman abuse. The voices of Kentucky women. *Violence Against Women, 1*(4), 309–38.

Weedon, C. (1987). *Feminist Practice and Poststructuralist Theory.* Oxford: Basil Blackwell.

Weisz, A. (2001). Spouse assault replication program: Studies of effects of arrest on domestic violence. *VAWnet Applied Research Documents.* Retrieved 11 September 2006, from http://www.vawnet. org/DomesticViolence/Research/VAWnetDocs/AR_arrest.php

Weldon, S. (2002). *Protest, Policy and the Problem of Violence Against Women, A Cross-National Comparison.* Pittsburgh: University of Pittsburgh Press.

Wescott, H. (1998). Disabled children and child protection. In C. Robinson and K. Stalker (eds), *Growing Up with Disability.* London: Jessica Kingsley.

Williams, C.R. (1996). *Identity, Difference and the 'Other'.* Unpublished PhD Thesis, University of Western Sydney, Campbelltown.

Williams, J. (2001). *Suicide and Attempted Suicide.* London: Penguin.

Williams, O., Boggess, J. and Carter, J. (2001). Fatherhood and domestic violence: Exploring the role of men who batter in the lives of their children. In S. Graham-Bermann and J. Edleson (eds), *Domestic Violence in the Lives of Children.* Washington: American Psychological Association.

Winsor, J. (2001). Workplace bullying. *Aboriginal and Islander Health Worker Journal*, *25*(3), 4–9.

Winsor-Dahlstrom, J. (2000). *Aboriginal Health Workers: Role, Recognition, Racism and Horizontal Violence in the Workplace*. The University of Sydney, Sydney.

Wittner, J. (1998). Reconceptualizing agency in domestic violence court. In N.A. Naples (ed.), *Community Activism and Feminist Politics: Organizing Across Race, Class, and Gender* (pp. 81–104). New York: Routledge.

Wolfe, V.V., Gentile, C. and Wolfe, D.A. (1989). The impact of sexual abuse on children: A PTSD formulation. *Behaviour Therapy*, *20*(2), 215–88.

Wolkind, S. and Rutter, M. (1984). Separation, loss and family relationships. In M. Rutter and L. Hersov (eds), *Child and Adolescent Psychiatry: Modern Approaches* (2nd edn). London: Blackwell Scientific Publications.

World Bank. (2005). *World Development Indicators 05: Reducing Poverty and Hunger*.

World Health Organization (WHO). (2001). World Health Organization Fact Sheet No. 128. Retrieved 21 November 2006.

World Health Organization (WHO). (2002). *The World Health Report 2002: Reducing Risks, Promoting Healthy Life*. Geneva: World Health Organization.

World Health Organization (WHO). (2005). *Multi-country Study on Women's Health and Domestic Violence against Women*. Geneva: World Health Organization.

World Health Organization (WHO). (2006a). Suicide rates per 100,000 by country, year and sex (Table). Retrieved 13 December 2006, from http://www.who.int/mental_health/prevention/suicide_ rates/en/index.html

World Health Organization (WHO). (2006b). Suicide prevention and special programmes. Retrieved 13 December 2006, from http://www.who.int/mental_health/prevention/suicide/suicideprevent/ en/index.html

World Health Organization (WHO) and The International Network for the Prevention of Elder Abuse (INPEA). (2002). *Missing Voices. Views of Older Persons on Elder Abuse*. Geneva: World Health Organization.

World Health Organization (WHO) & International Society for Prevention of Child Abuse and Neglect (ISPCAN). (2006). *Preventing Child Maltreatment: A Guide to Taking Action and Generating Evidence*. World Health Organization & International Society for Prevention of Child Abuse and Neglect.

Yip, P.S.F., Fu, K.W., Yang, K.C.T., Ip, B.Y.T., Chan, C.L.W. and Chen, E.Y.H. (2006). The effects of a celebrity suicide on suicide rates in Hong Kong. *Journal of Affective Disorders*, *93*(1–3), 245–52.

Yokota, K. (2006, 13 October). *Abuse and Violence Among Intimate Family Members*. Paper presented at the Symposium on Domestic Violence – Welfare of Children and Families, Baptist University Hong Kong.

Yoshihama, M. (2002). Policies and Services Addressing Domestic Violence in Japan: From Non-interference to Incremental Changes. *Women's Studies International Forum*, *25*, 541–53.

Young, I.R. (2003). The logic of masculinist protection: Reflections on the current security state. *Signs: Journal of Women and Culture*, *29*(1), 2–25.

Zussman, R. (1992). *Intensive Care: Medical Ethics and the Medical Profession*. Chicago: University of Chicago Press.

Index